# HYPOSPADIAS
## A GUIDE TO TREATMENT

The definitive guide for parents
with boys born with hypospadias.

Matt Dorow   |   Dr. Suzan Carmichael   |   Dr. Bill Kennedy
Genevieve Kilman   |   Ed Weaver Jr.

*ISBN: 1475088973*
*ISBN-13: 9781475088977*
*Library of Congress Control Number: 2012905637*
*CreateSpace, North Charleston, South Carolina*

This book would not have been possible without the enthusiastic support of so many people.

They all deserve thanks and praise.

Dr Bill Kennedy, Dr Suzan Carmichael, Genevieve Kilman and Ed Weaver, the co-authors, worked tirelessly through many revisions to complete their contributions. Betsy Miller gave us phenomenal editing guidance and helped us pull it all together. The Hypospadias and Epispadias Association Inc's members and board put on the excellent annual conference that brought us together as a group and allowed this information to be generated. Kelly Carter created the drawings, quickly and well. CreateSpace helped us get this book published, painlessly.

# Contents

# Prologue

*By Matt Dorow*

When our son was born, after the nurse had examined him, she presented him back to my wife and me and said: "Congratulations. Your son is healthy. He also has hypospadias. It is not a health concern. It is simply cosmetic and can be corrected later with surgery."

My wife and I were so happy that our son was healthy that these words of hypospadias went in one ear and out the other. Later, of course, those words began to ring louder and louder, and we determined to educate ourselves as much as possible as to what they meant. We turned to the internet and medical professionals for information. As a parent of a child with hypospadias, you have likely done the same. And you have likely had a similar experience to what we had. Some basic information came very quickly. You likely found out the same basics that we did:

Hypospadias, in its simplest terms, is when the urethral tube (where the urine flows) does not develop all the way to the end of the penis. Instead it terminates somewhere along the underside of the penis. Where the urethral tube terminates is where the urethral opening is located, and thus where the urine comes out (i.e., the pee hole). Where this urethral opening is determines the severity of the hypospadias. If the functioning urethral opening ends somewhere on the head of the penis, the case is considered mild, because the urine still shoots relatively forward, and the boy will be able to stand at a urinal. If the urethral opening is located on the shaft of the penis, then the condition is considered moderate (or severe if it is located at the very base of the penis), because the urine shoots downward, and the boy will therefore have to sit to urinate.

Hypospadias is one of the most common birth defects, affecting 4 to 6 per 1,000 boys. That means that approximately 600-900,000 American males today were born with the condition.

Hypospadias is not a life-threatening medical condition, but rather a functional one that can have psychological ramifications. Boys with moderate to severe hypospadias can become very self-conscious about their penises. Typical situations that provoke anxiety are having to sit to urinate, and concern that any sex partner they engage with will clearly see the difference in their penis.

Decisions about when and if to have surgery are highly personal and depend on the individual child's situation. Families should explain hypospadias to boys and help them accept themselves as they are. The goal is to avoid a situation in which a boy becomes so worried about being discovered that, during puberty, he develops obsessions or phobias regarding sexuality or sexual intimacy.

Surgical repair for hypospadias is now quite common and usually successful when performed by a top surgeon. However, there is very little information available about who the top surgeons in the world are, and what their success rates are.

And that is the sum of the basic information that we were able to find on the internet and talking to the medical professionals that we had access to. Beyond this basic information, there was nothing. There was not a single book written on the subject (other than highly technical medical journals).

Through massive persistence, we were able to gather bits and pieces of information by speaking to surgeons and nurses and getting referrals to other parents. The best information that we got came from talking to other parents. But getting access to parents was a laborious and painful process. We still felt that we hadn't gotten enough good information and needed to meet more parents, but how?

We discovered that there is a Hypospadias and Epispadias Assocation (HEA) that has an annual conference. We called up the executive director who told us that he expected at least several parents would be at that year's conference (in October, 2010), as well as adult men with hypospadias and several medical professionals in the field. While the conference sounded very small, informal and more geared toward being a support group for adult men, I decided to go, thinking that it was our best chance to gather a lot of information in a short period of time. And that is exactly what it turned out to be.

In two days, I listened to medical professionals walk through all of the surgical options, complications from those procedures, and possible causes of the condition. I spoke with adult men who were able to clearly articulate the emotional trauma that they had suffered, exactly how this trauma had been caused, and how I as a parent could help prevent altogether this trauma in my own child. I spoke with parents who were able to tell me of post-operative care successes and failures that they had had, so that I could learn from their experiences. In two days I got all the information and comfort that my wife and I were looking for.

It was then that I realized that this same information needed to be transmitted to the many other parents out there who face this same issue. I asked each of the lecturers if they'd be willing to write down the content of their lecture for a book. They all eagerly agreed to do so. What you will read in the following pages is what they wrote. If you like what they have written, then I highly encourage you to attend the annual HEA conference, as you will get so much more information there.

# Chapter 1: Introduction

*By Matt Dorow*

## Takeaways

For me, this book has two critical takeaways:

1.  Hypospadias repair (especially for the moderate to severe cases) is extremely delicate and difficult, requiring great skill and experience not only by the surgeon but also by the entire surgical team. Therefore, I highly recommend that you take the time to find not a good surgeon and team, but the best surgeon and team. Having one major surgery is trauma enough for a child. You don't want your child to have to experience it several times.

2.  Telling your child that he was born with hypospadias is critical, even if (maybe, especially if) he has had successful hypospadias repair. New complications can arise again during teenage years, and if a child doesn't know that he was born with hypospadias, he may be very frightened by these complications, and too embarrassed to tell you about them. Almost all the adult men with hypospadias that I have met told me that their teenage years were filled with emotional trauma because they thought that they were "freaks", "alone", etc. Each one of them told me that all this trauma could have been avoided if their parents had just told them that:

a. they were born with hypospadias,
b. that it is quite common, and
c. if a new complication should arise, it can be repaired.

Some also suggested that I find other men/boys with hypospadias for my son to talk to, so that he would have living proof that he wasn't' alone and that others with the condition are perfectly normal people. If the solution to avoiding emotional trauma is that simple – simply telling my son that he was born with hypospadias – then I certainly plan on doing it. I hope that you do as well.

## Outline
This book is broken into chaptures on the following issues:
- Causes
- Treatment
- Care
- Adult Story
- Parent Story

I will give you some of the highlights of each of these chapters here in the introduction, plus there is a short summary at the beginning of each chapter, but I highly encourage you to read the entire chapters to get all the detail.

## Causes
What causes hypospadias? In short, we don't know. There have been some inconclusive studies that have shown potential links to environmental factors. The media has picked up on these studies and sensationalized them. But the reality is that we simply don't know what causes hypospadias. The studies either show conflicting results or the study groups are too small to be meaningful.

What we do know is that somewhere between 10 and 16 weeks of pregnancy, something interrupts normal development and the urethral tube does not fully extend into the end of the penis. What causes that interruption or why, we do not know.

We also know that there is a genetic link. If a parent or a sibling has hypospadias, then the chances of another child being born with hypospadias will triple to about 1 in 50 (some sources say the rate jumps to 1 in 6). But beyond those small bits of knowledge, we do not know what causes hypospadias or why. Clearly more research is needed.

For me, the takeaway is that if you have a child born with hypospadias, know that this occurrence is likely not caused by anything that you did. In addition, if you want to have more children, do so. Hypospadias is not a physically painful or life-threatening condition, and it is much more likely that your future children will be born without it than with it.

**Treatment**

The goal of surgical hypospadias repair is to construct a urethral tube that terminates at the end of the penis. If the tube already terminates on the lower part of the penis head, then the tube is close enough to its final destination that the surgeon can simply peel back the outer skin, grab the existing urethral tube, stretch it to the end of the penis, and then stitch the outer skin back in place. This process is quite straightforward and has a very high success rate.

Repairing a moderate or severe case, where the urethral tube terminates on the underside of the penis shaft, however, is much more complicated. Because the tube is not close enough to its final destination, it cannot be stretched far enough to make it all the way to the tip of the penis. Therefore, an entirely new urethral tube must be crafted. The urethral skin is used to create a new urethral tube, which is then placed back into the penis, and the outer skin is folded back over the new urethral tube.

The two most common complications from these surgeries are fistulas and constrictions.

- Fistulas. After surgery, blood vessels must form from the surrounding flesh to the new urethral tube and sutured outer skin. If these blood vessels do not form at any point, then the flesh at that point will die, causing a hole, called a fistula, to develop. While a fistula is a new hole that is unrelated to the original urethral opening, pee will still come out of the fistula (and now also the urethral opening at the end of the penis) causing the boy to still have to sit to pee.
- Constrictions, also called "meatal stenosis". Scar tissue may form inside or at the end of the urethral tube, constricting the flow of urine. The result of this constriction can be either obvious (pee shooting to off in a direction, often up), or subtle (taking a longer time to urinate).

The repairs for both of these complications can often be straightforward.

Fistula repair is often merely a matter of removing the dead skin from around the fistula and grafting a patch of healthy skin onto the area. If, however, the fistula is on or near the glans (head of the penis) and therefore close to the correct urethral opening, then there may not be enough healthy skin left between the two holes to support a graft. In this case, the urethral tube may need to be created again, which is effectively a complete redo of a moderate to severe hypospadias surgery.

Constriction repair is almost always straightforward. It is usually an in-office procedure where the doctor dilates the urethra and applies topical corticosteroid ointment. If the constriction is severe, a minor surgery may be required, but this surgery won't be performed until at least 6 months after the initial operation, so that the existing tissue has first had a chance to fully heal.

## Care

This section provides advice on how to best navigate the medical system, including pre-operative and post-operative care, selecting a surgeon, longer-term care, emotional care and legal rights.

## Adult story

This section is written from the point of view of Ed Weaver Jr., a member of the Hypospadias and Epispadias Association (HEA) who was born with severe hypospadias. As a child he went through numerous surgeries without the benefit of information about hypospadias. He now advocates for providing accurate medical information about hypospadias and encourages families to have open discussions with their sons.

## Parent Story

This section describes my point of view as a parent of a son who was born with hypospadias. I present the challenges faced by parents and cover not only my own experience, but also what I've learned from physicians, other parents, and adults who were treated for hypospadias.

## Post-Operative Care Guide

This is an example of a post-operative care guide that is given to parents when their son goes home after surgery for hypospadias.

# Chapter 2: What Causes Hypospadias

*By Dr. Suzan Carmichael*

**Summary**

We do not yet know what causes hypospadias. We have some clues, and there are certainly some factors that seem to be associated with increased risk, but none of the studies to date have been conclusive. What follows is a summary of those studies, and where we need to look from here.

Since we don't really know what causes hypospadias, we can't make solid recommendations on what parents can do to reduce their risk of having a son with hypospadias. We do know that risk increases if there is a family history of hypospadias, such as in the father or in a previous son. But even then, it's important to keep in mind that if there is increased risk—based on family history or any of the other factors discussed below—it is much more likely that a baby will be born without hypospadias than with it!

**Background**

Hypospadias occurs when the urethra does not close correctly. Instead of opening at the tip of the penis, it opens somewhere on the underside. The opening can range from being a little off center to being in the scrotal or perineal area ( between the scrotum and penis). The term comes from the Greek "hypo," which means under, and "spadon," which means a rip or opening [1].

## Normal Male Genitalia

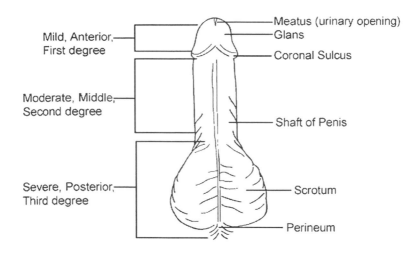

Figure 1: *Illustration of penis, including location of meatus in mild, moderate and severe hypospadias. (Source: Kelly Carter)*

Normal urethral closure occurs during the $10^{th}$-$16^{th}$ weeks of pregnancy. It depends on androgens (e.g., testosterone) produced by the fetal testis. It can be induced in laboratory animals by treatment with chemicals that interfere with androgen synthesis and function, including estrogens. Therefore, it is thought that in humans, hypospadias is probably caused by environmental and genetic factors that impair maternal, fetal, or placental androgen and estrogen metabolism. In most cases, some combination of environmental and/or genetic factors that would not cause hypospadias on their own probably interact and thus result in hypospadias. This knowledge provides a helpful framework for looking for causes, but our actual understanding of what causes hypospadias in humans is relatively limited, and it could certainly extend beyond exposures related to androgen function.

This chapter reviews what we know about causes of hypospadias and what types of factors are associated with increased risk. The studies that are the basis of our knowledge about risk factors tend to be from the field of epidemiology, meaning that they observed what factors were associated with risk of hypospadias at the population level. Such findings can suggest what may be associated with increased risk, but they typically cannot tell us what caused hypospadias in a particular individual. To consider whether or how findings from these studies can help pinpoint what may have caused hypospadias in an individual, one would need to consult a genetic counselor or medical geneticist.

## Prevalence and Trends

There are approximately four to six cases of hypospadias per 1,000 male births. Prevalences reported by specific studies are sometimes much lower or higher than this average, sometimes due to real differences, and sometimes simply due to limitations in how well the studies were conducted. Regardless, it is clear that hypospadias is one of the most common structural birth defects.

Concerns about an increase in the prevalence of hypospadias over time are often stated in the scientific literature. Studies have suggested increases especially in the 1980's and 1990's in some countries, including the U.S., but more recent studies tend to suggest that the prevalence is holding steady. The potentially increasing prevalence has often been cited as evidence that harmful environmental exposures cause hypospadias. However, as noted, it's debatable whether prevalences really are increasing. Furthermore, even if environmental exposures do cause hypospadias, we don't know which ones are the culprits, much less whether or not exposure to them has been increasing. So, we're still pretty close to square one, not really knowing what causes hypospadias, but there are some interesting clues.

**Risk Factors**

Although the exact number is hard to pinpoint, probably less than 10 percent of cases can be explained by known causes such as specific endocrine abnormalities or genetic defects. It is important to rule these causes out in individuals, though, because they may affect plans for treatment and follow-up over time. In most cases, the cause of hypospadias is unknown. Many factors are associated with increased risk of hypospadias, although the evidence is too limited to say they 'cause' hypospadias at this point. This section provides a summary of these factors.

Maternal and infant characteristics. Several maternal characteristics are associated with increased risk of hypospadias: older age, being overweight, Caucasian race-ethnicity, and higher socioeconomic status. Several studies have evaluated smoking, and results do not suggest a strong association. Maternal alcohol consumption and use of illicit drugs have not been well-evaluated. One of the most consistent infant characteristics associated with hypospadias is intra-uterine growth retardation, meaning that babies with hypospadias are often smaller than expected, given their gestational age at delivery. First-born babies are also more likely to have hypospadias.

Placental insufficiency. The placenta plays a critical role in controlling fetal synthesis of androgens and estrogens, and it is becoming fully functional at the same time the urethra begins to develop. Therefore, early compromised placental function is often suggested as a contributor to hypospadias risk. This idea is supported by the fact that hypospadias is associated with several indicators of poor placental function, including intrauterine growth retardation, pre-eclampsia, and having a twin pregnancy. Some studies have also shown hypospadias to be associated with actual indicators of compromised placental function.

Nutrition. Some nutrients are associated with estrogen and androgen synthesis or metabolism, the most well-known being phytoestrogens. One study indicated that the phytoestrogen genistein, which is particularly high in soy products, could induce hypospadias in animals experimentally [2]. One small epidemiologic study suggested that a vegetarian diet and high intake of legumes (which are high in lignans, a grouping of phytoestrogens) were associated with increased risk of hypospadias [3]. This study has been cited repeatedly in the literature to provide evidence that an estrogenic exposure may cause hypospadias; this statement rests on the assumption that vegetarians had higher intake of estrogenic nutrients like phytoestrogens. However, several subsequent studies have not confirmed an association with vegetarianism or intake of soy protein or lignans. Given limitations such as small sample sizes and incomplete dietary assessment, however, all of these studies are somewhat problematic for drawing meaningful conclusions.

Maternal intake of multivitamin or mineral supplements, especially products containing folic acid, has been associated with reduced risk of several birth defects, most notably neural tube defects like spina bifida. Studies have not demonstrated that supplements are protective against hypospadias, although of course it is important to take them for other health benefits during pregnancy.

Sex hormone medications, fertility, and fertility treatments. Sex hormone medications that may be taken during early pregnancy primarily include progestins (natural progesterone and synthetic progesterone and testosterone derivatives that produce biologic effects similar to those of progesterone). It has been hypothesized that progestins may increase hypospadias risk by interfering with the production or action of fetal androgens. The formulations and doses of these types of medications have changed substantially in the past few decades. One class of progestins—oral contraceptives—do not appear to be associated with hypospadias.

Two studies that are relatively recent—and therefore more relevant to today's exposures—have observed at least a two-fold increase in risk of hypospadias among women who took progestins for the purpose of preventing pregnancy loss or complications [4,5]. Limitations of these studies include their reliance on maternal recall of exposures and lack of information on the specific formulation of the medication (there are synthetic and natural forms) and dose.

Some studies have also suggested that maternal or paternal sub-fertility or fertility-related procedures are associated with hypospadias, but it is uncertain whether the findings are due to underlying medical conditions or fertility-related procedures or medications.

Diethylstilbestrol (DES) is a synthetic estrogen that was widely prescribed several decades ago but no longer in use. A few studies have examined whether hypospadias is increased among women who were exposed *in utero* (in other words, when their mothers were pregnant with them) to DES. The first study suggested a 20-fold increased risk; it was restricted to women with fertility problems [6]. Subsequent studies reported no association or more modest associations. The study reporting no association was the only one that had actual medical record information on maternal DES exposure *in utero*. The other studies relied on maternal recall, which may be more subject to errors. Although the results are intriguing from a scientific point of view, pregnancies among women who were exposed *in utero* to DES are currently quite rare.

Other medications. Corticosteroids (glucocorticoids) inhibit placental development and fetal synthesis of androgen precursors. They have anti-inflammatory and immune system suppressing properties that make them useful in the treatment of a variety of conditions, including asthma, rheumatoid arthritis, allergic reactions and eczema. An experimental animal study indicated that giving the corticosteroid prednisone to pregnant rats resulted in hypospadias in their offspring, but in humans, maternal corticosteroid use has not been associated with hypospadias.

Loratadine is an over-the-counter anti-histamine. It was associated with increased risk of hypospadias in one study, but subsequent studies have not confirmed this finding.

Valproic acid, which is primarily used as an anti-convulsant, is contraindicated (not recommended) during pregnancy due to its association with birth defects, including hypospadias.

Environmental contaminants. There is extensive public concern that environmental contaminants may be disrupting endocrine (hormonal) function in humans. Such contaminants are often called 'endocrine disruptors.' Some of the more familiar endocrine disruptors include, for example, phthalates and BPA (bisphenol-A), which may be found in products such as plastic baby bottles and toys. Some endocrine disruptors have estrogenic effects (in other words, they have some of the same functions as estrogens), which may in turn inhibit androgens like testosterone. For this reason, there is concern that they may be associated with increased risk of hypospadias. Although this concern is stated repeatedly, there are unfortunately few rigorous studies that directly evaluate whether environmental contaminants are associated with increased risk of hypospadias.

Many widely used agricultural pesticides are potential endocrine disruptors, and some of them can induce hypospadias in experimental animal studies. A few studies have examined maternal serum levels of the pesticide DDT (dichlorodiphenyltrichloroethane) and its metabolite DDE, which were used until the 1970s but remain in the environment. The studies reported minimal to no association with hypospadias.

A number of studies have used parental occupations as proxies for exposure to pesticides or other potential endocrine disruptors. A recent review concluded that parental occupations likely to involve pesticide exposure may be associated with slightly increased risk (20-40%) [7]. Results related to other types of occupations or exposures have largely been conflicting.

One of the biggest challenges in this area is getting good measures of exposures. As noted, only a few studies have directly measured exposures (for example, in serum). They have tended to examine one compound at a time. Studies of mixtures of exposures may be important, especially if the effects of chemicals in combination outweigh the effects of each chemical in isolation. Functional consequences of these types of exposures are not well understood, although ultimately it is the functional consequence that would be of interest as a cause of hypospadias.

In summary, although a variety of exposures related to maternal, fetal and placental endocrine function have been *proposed* to cause hypospadias, their association with hypospadias in humans remains uncertain.

Risk factors by hypospadias severity. A common question is whether the risk factors for hypospadias are the same regardless of severity. As noted, hypospadias can involve the urethral opening being just a little bit off-center, to being located closer to the scrotum or perineum. Most studies group all cases together, regardless of the location of the opening. Sometimes this is because studies do not have information on the location of the opening, and sometimes it is because their numbers are too small to be able to split them up into separate analyses. Other studies may be totally restricted to more severe cases (such as the opening is on the penile shaft or at the scrotum). There has been some thought that the urethra forms by a somewhat different process in the glanular area (the tip) than further down, although more recent theories support a more similar process for the entire urethra. This leads to some concern that the causes of hypospadias may be different, depending on how severe the case. At this point, the issue remains debatable.

Association of hypospadias with other reproductive health outcomes. Hypospadias co-occurs more often than expected with other outcomes related to male reproductive health, including cryptorchidism (undescended testes), poor semen quality, and testicular cancer. Sometimes this clustering of outcomes is referred to as the testicular dysgenesis syndrome. The idea is that since they co-occur, they may share some common causes, especially causes that may have their impacts during fetal development (during pregnancy). Regardless of whether or not a common cause is eventually uncovered for these outcomes, for families affected by hypospadias it is probably most important to keep in mind that testicular cancer is very rare and that the majority of cases of hypospadias do not have impaired semen quality [8].

## Genetic Susceptibility

Genetics undoubtedly contribute to hypospadias. Studies that examine recurrence within families indicate that risk of hypospadias is increased several-fold in male siblings, sons and other close relatives, and that these risks may be transmitted similarly through the maternal and paternal sides of the family [9]. Most studies suggest that the more severe the case, the more likely is familial recurrence. However, reported recurrence risks for mild cases could be underestimated because of under-reporting. Evidence for a contribution of genetics also comes from animal studies showing that hypospadias can be caused by manipulating the action of certain genes and from human studies showing that single genes can cause syndromes that include hypospadias. In general, the evidence points to the causes of hypospadias as being "multifactorial," meaning that small effects of many genes and/or environmental factors act in concert to affect risk [10,11].

As with environmental exposures, our understanding of which genes may affect hypospadias risk is limited. With improvements in genetic technology, it is hoped that substantial gains in knowledge will emerge over the next several years.

Most studies have focused on genes that affect the development of the genital tubercle, which is the precursor to the penis, and genes that affect sex steroid hormone synthesis or metabolism [12]. Certain genes are associated with syndromes, but as noted earlier, most hypospadias cases are non-syndromic. Some of the more likely candidates among non-syndromic cases include *SRD5A2* (5a-reductase type II), which converts testosterone to dihydrotestosterone in the developing urethra; *AR* (androgen receptor), *ESR1* and *ESR2* (estrogen receptors), which regulate the action of androgens and estrogens, respectively; *ATF3* (activating transcription factor 3), which interacts with the estrogen receptor; and *MAMLD1* (mastermind-like domain containing 1, or *CXorf6*), which affects testosterone production. It is difficult to estimate the percentage of cases that are affected by mutations in these genes or other genes from these pathways, because studies have varied considerably in many ways. For example, some studies may examine mutations at only one or a couple of sites in the gene, which provides incomplete information. Other studies may include a mix of syndromic and non-syndromic cases, which makes it difficult to generalize.

The first genome-wide association study of hypospadias was published recently [13]. These types of studies examine large numbers of mutations across many different genes, in hopes of discovering new genes that may contribute to an outcome. This study's strongest findings were for a gene called *DGKK*, which had not previously been examined in relation to hypospadias. Mutations in the gene were present in about 50% of the cases, but also in about one-third of the comparison group, which did not have hypospadias. Having a mutation in the gene was associated with a two- to three-fold increased risk of hypospadias. This finding needs to be examined in other study populations to determine its true relevance.

In general, the current literature on genes and hypospadias is somewhat piecemeal. Most studies are relatively small, examine one gene at a time, and have not been replicated (a finding is much stronger if it can be replicated across multiple studies, versus only being shown in one study). Studies that investigate interactions among multiple genes, as well as interactions of genes with environmental exposures, will be critical to moving our understanding forward. This approach fits with the 'multifactorial' model described above. Recent advances in genetic technologies should make conducting these more complex types of studies more affordable. Studying interactions makes biologic sense because many genes act together to regulate genital tubercle development and urethral closure. Similarly, certain genes may impact the effects of environmental exposures; for example, the negative impact of a pesticide on testosterone production may be worse in a person who has a gene variant that disrupts his or her ability to break down pesticides or make testosterone.

It is hoped that eventually, our knowledge in this area will be solid enough to enable genetic screening to identify who is at high risk of having a baby with hypospadias. This type of knowledge can help clinicians improve treatment plans, it can help scientists figure out what causes an outcome, and it can help families understand what might have caused hypospadias in their son and refine how high the risk is for future sons.

## Advice on How to Interpret the Literature Yourself

The web has transformed access to information, including scientific articles. Interpreting a body of literature (or even a single article) is difficult even for someone who is well-trained to do it. Many factors go into it, such as being able to judge the quality of study designs, how well exposures were measured, whether appropriate analytic techniques were used, and whether final interpretations really reflect the actual results. It is especially difficult to synthesize findings when so many of them conflict with each other. Having strong pre-conceived notions about associations can bias one's interpretation of the literature. One important point to keep in mind is that rarely can a single study stand on its own; findings are much more likely to be valid if they are observed repeatedly across multiple study populations. An additional few rules of thumb are that the larger the study, the easier it is to get precise estimates of associations; the more representative the study group is of the underlying population, the more likely its associations are applicable to the general population (for instance, if only a small percentage of eligible subjects participated, the results may not apply to the general population); and it is important to pay as much attention to negative findings (studies that do not find an association) as to positive findings. It is also important to keep in mind the context. Most of the risk factors discussed above increase risk only modestly, typically around within 1.5- to 2-fold times the usual prevalence. So, even when faced with these possible risk factors, the risk of having a baby without hypospadias is much greater than the risk of having one with it. And for infants who are born with hypospadias, fortunately, treatment options are continually improving, as described in the next chapter.

## References

1. Bremer JL. Hypospadias and epispadias: A philological note. *New Engl J Med.* 1932;207(12):537-539.

2. Vilela ML, Willingham E, Buckley J, et al. Endocrine disruptors and hypospadias: role of genistein and the fungicide vinclozolin. *Urology.* 2007;70(3):618-621.

3. North K, Golding J. A maternal vegetarian diet in pregnancy is associated with hypospadias. The ALSPAC Study Team. Avon Longitudinal Study of Pregnancy and Childhood. *BJU Int.* 2000;85:107-113.

4. Carmichael SL, Shaw GM, Laurent C, et al. Maternal progestin intake and risk of hypospadias. *Arch Pediatr Adolesc Med.* 2005;159:957-962.

5. Kallen B, Martinez-Frias ML, Castilla EE, Robert E, Lancaster PAL, et al. Hormone therapy during pregnancy

and isolated hypospadias: an international case-control study. *Int J Risk Safety Med.* 1992;3:183-198.

6.  Klip H, Verloop J, van Gool JD, Koster ME, Burger CW, van Leeuwen FE. Hypospadias in sons of women exposed to diethylstilbestrol in utero: a cohort study. *Lancet.* 2002;359(9312):1102-1107.

7.  Rocheleau CM, Romitti PA, Dennis LK. Pesticides and hypospadias: a meta-analysis. *J Pediatr Urol.* Feb 2009;5(1):17-24.

8.  Asklund C, Jensen TK, Main KM, Sobotka T, Skakkebaek NE, Jorgensen N. Semen quality, reproductive hormones and fertility of men operated for hypospadias. *Int J Androl.* Feb 2010;33(1):80-87.

9.  Schnack TH, Zdravkovic S, Myrup C, et al. Familial aggregation of hypospadias: a cohort study. *Am J Epidemiol.* Feb 1 2008;167(3):251-256.

10. Harris EL. Genetic epidemiology of hypospadias. *Epidemiol Rev.* 1990;12:29-40.

11. Opitz JM. Hypospadias [editorial comment]. *Am J Med Genet.* 1985;21:57-60.

12. Kojima Y, Kohri K, Hayashi Y. Genetic pathway of external genitalia formation and molecular etiology of hypospadias. *J Pediatr Urol.* Aug 2010;6(4):346-354.

13. van der Zanden LF, van Rooij IA, Feitz WF, et al. Common variants in DGKK are strongly associated with risk of hypospadias. *Nat Genet.* Jan 2010;43(1):48-50.

# Chapter 3: Treatment of Hypospadias

*By Dr. Bill Kennedy*

**Summary**

In this chapter, Dr. Kennedy provides background information about urethral development and reviews the various surgical techniques used to repair differing severity levels of hypospadias, along with common post-operative care and complications that may occur. The key take-away here is that surgical repair of moderate and severe hypospadias is a very delicate and challenging surgery. Complication rates are significant.

**Urethral Development**

Hypospadias is the failure of the urethra (urine tube) to close completely on the underside (hypo) of the shaft of the penis. This should be differentiated from the related, but developmentally very distinct problem of epispadias, where the urethra is open on the upside (epi) of the penis. Epispadias is a very significant birth defect that is often associated with exstrophy of the bladder. The problems of epispadias and bladder exstrophy will not be discussed in this chapter as they require a very different approach to repair.

When the penis has formed correctly during pregnancy, the average length is 2.5 cm (+0.7 cm) and the average diameter (width) is 1.1 cm (+0.2 cm). The penis will usually have a slight increase in growth around 3 months of age when the Leydig cells in the boy's testis produce a surge of testosterone. This growth is helpful if surgical repair is to be considered by the parents.

With hypospadias, the urethral opening can be located anywhere from the point just below the scrotum (sac which contains the testicles) all the way to a point just below the usual position on the glans (head) of the penis. The opening is usually located directly in the middle of the structure on what appears to be a seam in the penis and scrotum. This seam has a medical name called the median raphe. It is the place at which the two halves of the penis and scrotum fuse together. The closure of the urinary tube (urethra) begins at the point just below the scrotum and closes much like a zipper would from the base (bottom) to the apex (top) of the penis. There may sometimes appear to be more than one opening for the urethra along this line, but only one of these openings is the true urethral meatus (opening) through which the urine will flow. If you observe your son carefully, the lowest of the openings is always the one through which the urine flows. Often times parents may believe that there are two openings, one at the very top (apex) of the glans and another located lower along the median raphe. The opening at the apex is not a true opening and represents the ectodermal intrusion or ectodermal pit (see Figure 2.) that occurs during development of the penis. When the penis forms completely, the ectodermal intrusion joins the urethra that is zipping up from below, to form the natural opening at the tip of the penis.

Fig. 2

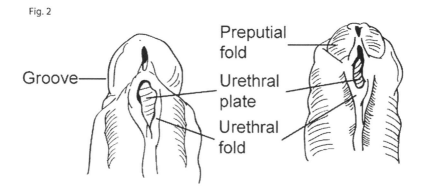

*Figure 2: The underside of the penis during early pregnancy, closure of the urethra. (Source: Kelly Carter)*

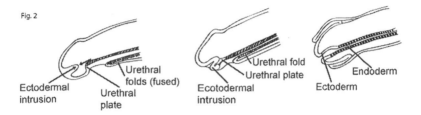

Fig. 2

Ectodermal intrusion

Urethral plate

Urethral folds (fused)

Ecotodermal intrusion

Urethral fold

Urethral plate

Endoderm

Ectoderm

*Figure 3: Side view of the penis in early pregnancy demonstrating the closure of the urethra from the base (bottom) towards the apex (top). (Source: Kelly Carter)*

## Hypospadias Classification

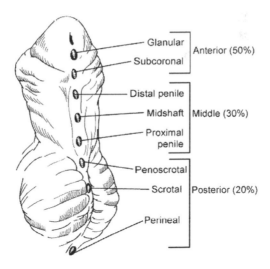

Glanular

Subcoronal

Anterior (50%)

Distal penile

Midshaft

Middle (30%)

Proximal penile

Penoscrotal

Scrotal

Posterior (20%)

Perineal

*Figure 4: Underside of the penis, possible locations for the true urethral meatus. The names to the side are often used in describing the magnitude of the child's hypospadias. (Source: Kelly Carter)*

The meatal opening of the penis can be divided into three categories: 1) anterior, 2) middle, and 3) posterior. Anterior refers to the glanular and subcoronal locations. It accounts for approximately 50% of all hypospadias. Middle refers to the distal penile, midshaft and proximal penile locations. It accounts for approximately 30% of all hypospadias. Finally, posterior refers to the penoscrotal, scrotal and perineal locations. They account for approximately 20% of all hypospadias.

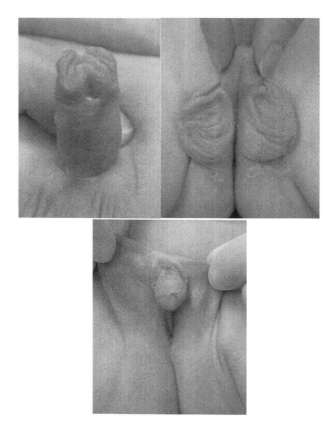

*Figure 5: A) Example of patient with anterior or subcoronal hypospadias. B) Example of patient with middle or posterior shaft hypospadias and bifid scrotum. C) Example of patient with posterior or perineal hypospadias. (Source: Dr Bill Kennedy)*

## Elements of Hypospadias

If we carefully look at a boy born with hypospadias, we will find that there are several components. It is important to understand these components as each will play a role in a family's decision as to whether surgical repair is desired.

## Foreskin

In the vast majority of hypospadias, the foreskin is incompletely fused (joined) on the underside of the penis. This leads to the foreskin appearing draped over the top side of the head of the penis. This appearance is called the "dorsal hood." Often times a health care provider not familiar with hypospadias may even inform a parent that their son was born "partially circumcised" and therefore no circumcision needs to be performed. In fact, they are "partially" correct in that if any abnormality of the penis is identified at birth, it is best not to allow anyone but a specialist to make the determination if a circumcision can be safely performed. The terminology "partially circumcised" is not correct, as no procedure or traumatic event has occurred to the child to injure or remove a portion of the foreskin—it has just failed to fuse!

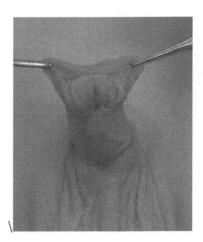

*Figure 6: Example of dorsal hooded foreskin in a boy with distal shaft hypospadias. (Source: Dr Bill Kennedy)*

On rare occasions the foreskin can completely fuse, thereby concealing an anterior hypospadias completely contained within the glans of the penis. This variant of hypospadias may not be identified at the time of birth or even in advance of a parent requesting that their son be circumcised. This variant of hypospadias is often referred to as an "MIP" variant of hypospadias. MIP is an acronym which refers to Megameatus Intact Prepuce. Megameatus refers to the hypospadiac opening in the glans, which is slightly larger (mega) than normal. Intact prepuce refers to the foreskin being completely fused. A physician performing a circumcision on a child without identifying this rare variant of hypospadias in advance has not harmed the child or prevented a successful hypospadias repair from being done at a future date. Families in which circumcision is not part of their tradition may never be aware that their child has a minor form of hypospadias in the case of the MIP variant.

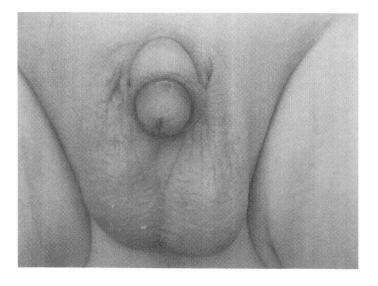

*Figure 7a: A boy born with MIP who had routine circumcision performed at birth. (Source: Dr Bill Kennedy)*

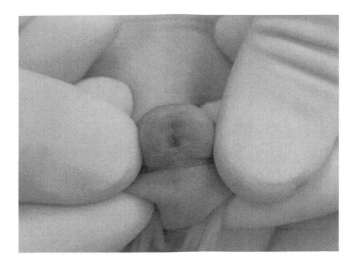

*Figure 7b: Close up view of boy born with MIP who had routine circumcision performed at birth. Notice the appearance of "two" meatal openings. The upper dimple is the "ectodermal pit" and the lower opening is the true meatus through which all urine flows. (Source: Dr Bill Kennedy)*

## Urethral Meatus

This is the heart of the hypospadias anomaly. It refers to where the actual opening of the urethra is positioned. The medical term "dystopia" is used to describe that the urethral opening is positioned away from the tip of the penis. Frequently the opening may appear to be close to the top of the penis, but at the time of surgery, the pediatric urologist may find that it extends further down the shaft of the penis, creating a larger defect to correct. This may occur for two reasons:

1) The upper portion of the urethral tissue, although fused, is of very poor quality and needs to be discarded.

2) The curvature associated with the hypospadias is very severe.

Curvature or chordee will be discussed next. Figures 4 a-c portray the varying degrees of meatal dystopia associated with hypospadias.

**Chordee**

Chordee or penile curvature refers to a very important component of hypospadias. The degree of curvature can vary greatly. There may be no curvature and the penis may be completely straight. This is often the case in the MIP variant of hypospadias and is frequently the reason why a circumcision may be performed before the mild glanular hypospadias is identified. When chordee is present, it may range from mild to moderate and even severe.

Often the degree of hypospadias (incomplete urinary tube) correlates with the degree of chordee (penile curvature). So patients with anterior hypospadias tend to have mild chordee and others who have middle or posterior hypospadias tend to have moderate to severe chordee. Occasionally we can see a mild chordee with severe penoscrotal hypospadias or a mild hypospadias with a severe chordee. The curvature of the penis is often what gives the boy with hypospadias a penis that appears shorter than the average boy. The good news is that most chordee is easily corrected. In doing so, one can restore the penis to a more normal appearing length.

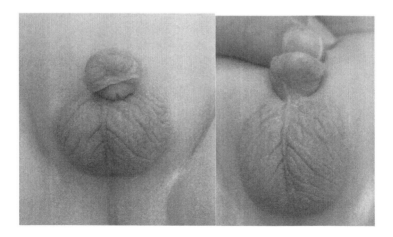

*Figure 8: A) Resting view of a boy with a moderate/severe 90 degree curvature of the penile shaft. B) Ventral (underside) view of same boy with moderate/severe chordee demonstrating the shortened penile length. (Source: Dr Bill Kennedy)*

Chordee can be caused by two distinct abnormalities at two different portions of the penile shaft anatomy. The most common reason is the deposition of inelastic fibrous tissue just under the fused skin of the penile shaft. The inelastic tissue on the undersurface of the penile shaft results in a downward curvature of the penis. This is depicted in Figure 8. More severe chordee can also result from a difference in the length of the corporal body (cylinders in the penile shaft that cause erections). If the upper side of the cylinder is longer than the bottom side of the cylinder, it will result in a downward curve of the penile shaft. The reason for understanding the difference between these two distinct causes of chordee is that they will determine strategies for surgical correction.

Figure 9 shows a cross sectional view of the penis (imagine you are slicing it like a loaf of french bread). The figure shows the corporal bodies, the intact urethra with the muscular wall supporting it, and the fascia (layers of tissue) holding all three structures together. Note the inelastic fibrous tissue, which causes most chordee.

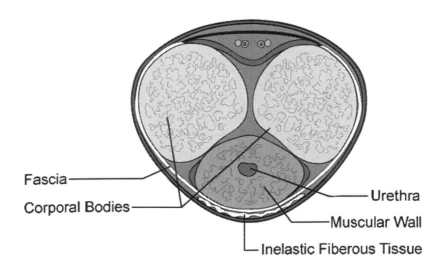

*Figure 9: Cross-sectional view of the penis. (Source: Kelly Carter)*

**Associated Urogenital Abnormalities**

There are other genital (non-penile) abnormalities that may be associated with hypospadias. These may also be discovered by your physician during a detailed examination of your child. These anomalies are undescended testis (UDT), inguinal hernia, hydrocele and/or utricle. UDT, hernias and hydroceles occur in association with hypospadias approximately 10% of the time. These three problems are also very common in newborn boys and may occur without hypospadias. Depending on the nature of the problem, the child may require surgery for these associated issues. If this is the case, then this should enter into the discussion of timing of an anticipated repair for the hypospadias. Very frequently UDTs and hydroceles may correct themselves and not require surgery.

Utricle (a pouch formed in the urethra) is an abnormality of the urethra much closer to the bladder and is often associated with difficulty in passing a catheter. Utricles are more common with the more severe forms of hypospadias and result from the under-virilization of the male anatomy. Utricles usually do not need surgical repair but are helpful to know about. As parents, you might find out about them as a result of difficulty of the physician in catheterizing your son or if x-rays of the urethra or cystoscopy (view of urethra through telescope) have been performed. If you know your son's urethra has a utricle, you should share this information with any health professional attempting to catheterize your son, as they may choose to modify their technique slightly to make it easier to insert the catheter.

**Decisions About Surgical Repair**

Now that you have learned about the possible causes of hypospadias and also understand the components of hypospadias, we can move on to the discussion of why parents and patients consider surgical repair. The good news is that hypospadias is rarely a "life threatening" condition. As a result, parents should not feel pressured to make any decisions about repair until they understand all the issues. The only time that hypospadias would be a truly emergent issue is if the urethral abnormality were such that it created retention of urine (inability for the boy to pee). In this situation, the health of the kidneys could be compromised requiring some urgent decisions. This is exceedingly rare, but physicians learn never to say "never" when it comes to the human body!

My general approach in discussing the reasons to consider surgical repair are broken down into four categories:

1. Direction of urinary stream
2. Erectile function
3. Fertility
4. Cosmetics

We'll explore these four categories in more detail

**Direction of Urine Stream**

Perhaps the most common functional impairment with hypospadias is the direction of the urinary stream. In a boy with normal penile anatomy, the urethral meatus is at the tip of the penis and therefore he can stand to urinate and aim the stream directly into the toilet. This may be a challenge for the boy born with hypospadias. Depending on the degree of hypospadias, the boy may be able to stand and void just as straight as any other. Conversely, the position of the urinary opening may be so far down the shaft of the penis that the boy must sit down to urinate. There may be a small degree of angulation of the urinary stream requiring the standing boy to mildly adjust his aim all the way to such severe angulation that it is impossible to get the stream directed into the toilet.

It is important for parents to understand that the diagnosis of hypospadias has NO impact on a boy's ability to potty train or his future urinary continence (that is, his ability to control *when* he pees). The portion of the male anatomy associated with urinary continence is located much closer to the bladder and is not affected by the portion of the urethra that has not closed. No matter how severe the hypospadias may appear, the boy will always be able to potty train. The only reasons for potty training not to occur would be if the child had an independent spinal cord problem (e.g., spina bifida) not related to the hypospadias or a developmental delay.

## Erectile Function

The issues associated with erectile function and hypospadias are a result of the component chordee and not the incomplete urethra. During early childhood, there is never a reason associated with chordee that warrants an urgent surgery. In fact a mild degree of chordee may never cause a boy any erectile dysfunction during his lifetime.

More severe chordee may become associated with: 1) discomfort or pain with erection or 2) inability to penetrate a partner during sexual intercourse. When boys go through puberty and their erectile function becomes more robust and sustained due to higher testosterone levels, the more pronounced curvatures associated with moderate to severe chordee may create pain. In the extreme cases of chordee, the curve of the penis may bend so sharply in the downward direction that vaginal penetration is not possible. Careful examination by an experienced pediatric urologist can often help guide the assessment and subsequent discussion with parents on the likelihood of these more significant impairments.

## Fertility

Fertility is perhaps the most difficult of these issues to discuss. To have a discussion most appropriate for your child, we should subdivide the boys into three groups: 1) boys with only hypospadias, 2) boys with associated testicular abnormalities, and 3) boys with genetic and chromosomal abnormalities.

In the first group of boys, which is the largest, there will be no issues with future fertility that are different from any other adult male. Although they may have hypospadias and/or chordee, the vast majority will have normal hormonal production at puberty and appropriate production of sperm. If the hypospadias and chordee are corrected or very mild, the adult male will likely have normal sexual intercourse with his partner and be able to inseminate her (get her pregnant) successfully. If the chordee prevents penetration or the uncorrected urethral opening is so far back on the penile shaft that the ejaculate (semen/sperm) cannot be deposited in the vaginal canal, then fertility will be impaired. In these situations, artificial insemination may assist in achieving a successful pregnancy. No matter how severe the initial hypospadias and chordee, if a successful repair has been achieved, then spontaneous pregnancy without assisted techniques should be possible.

In the group of boys with associated testicular problems, such as undescended testis and/or testicular dysgenesis (defective formation), there may be additional hurdles to fertility. This fertility impairment is independent of the hypospadias and chordee. It is associated with the abnormality of the testicle itself. Boys with chromosomal abnormalities and hypospadias may have fertility challenges due to the chromosomal disorder. Additional discussion of these issues is beyond the scope of this chapter, so please consult your medical professional for further information if they are of concern to you.

**Cosmetics**

Beauty is in the eye of the beholder! No matter how much we write about or discuss hypospadias, all patients, parents and physicians will never come to consensus on how to address the significance of cosmetics in this discussion. What is certain is that people have very passionate opinions. We must accept that each individual will assign a different priority to this aspect of the surgical repair. We should not pretend these concerns do not exist, but rather openly address and discuss them as part of the decision process. It is only through open discussion that patients and parents will be able to fully assess the role that surgical repair may have in their individual case.

## Introduction to Surgical Techniques for Hypospadias Repair

Once the patient or his parents have made a decision that surgery is the treatment of choice, then the conversation with their surgeon usually focuses on the possible techniques for the surgical repair. This conversation can often be overwhelming. Even additional personal research can be confusing as the sheer number and complex names of procedures can fill an entire chapter (See Table 1). I find it most productive for patients, parents and even surgeons in training to focus on the basic principles of the surgical repair, and then the topic becomes instantly manageable!

## Basic Principles of Chordee Repair

It is easiest to think about hypospadias surgery as being broken into two major parts. The first part is the correction of the chordee or penile curvature and the second part is the repair of the incomplete urinary tube (urethra).

To repair the chordee, the surgeon will determine at the time of the operation if the curvature results from the fibrous tissue just under the penile shaft skin or if it results from the unequal length of the top and bottom sides of the corporal bodies (the tubes that cause natural erections). In order to differentiate these two factors, an artificial erection is performed by the surgeon while the child is asleep in the operating room. The artificial erection can be done very safely and painlessly for the child at this time using injection of sterile fluid into the corporal body while a small tourniquet (a device to reduce the blood flow) is applied to the base of the penis. Some surgeons prefer to use a medication called alprostadil to achieve the same artificial erection if application of the tourniquet is made difficult due to penile length or severe degree of curvature. Either technique is performed after the initial mobilization (often called "degloving") of the penile shaft skin. The fibrous tissue is often completely removed at the time of mobilization of the skin. This will result in a nearly completely straight penis on artificial erection. No additional procedures are needed if this is the case.

In the event that the penis has residual curvature with the artificial erection, then a procedure to equalize the length of the corporal bodies is performed. The easiest way to equalize the corporal length is to perform a small excision or plication (similar to pleating) of the upper side of the corporal body. There are several ways to perform this technique and one example is demonstrated in figure 10. Here you can see the artificial erection technique being performed to show residual curvature and the plication procedure used to completely correct the residual chordee.

Fig. 5

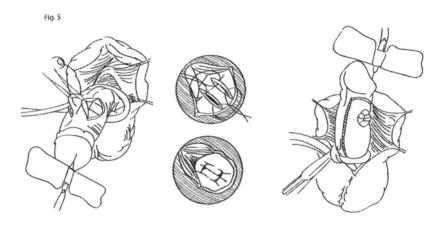

*Figure 10: A) Artificial erection and residual chordee. Plication of the upper part of the corporal bodies with permanent stitches. B) Straight penis on artificial erection after corporal plication. (Source: Kelly Carter)*

Another alternative exists to repairing chordee when the curvature is severe and the penile length is significantly below average. In these rare situations, a material may be grafted to the shorter underside of the corporal body to extend its length and straighten the penis. Originally, skin (dermal) grafts were used. Biomaterials have more recently become popular for this type of surgical procedure (see figure 11). Grafting procedures cannot be used to make the penile length any greater than the actual penile length. It is just an alternative to plication procedures, with a higher complication rate than the former.

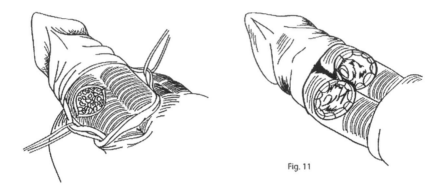

Fig. 11

*Figure 11: A) Incision made in the underside of the corporal body. B) Dermal grafts inserted and sutured in place on both corporal bodies. (Source: Kelly Carter)*

## Basic Principles of Urethral Reconstruction

Once chordee has been adequately corrected in the first portion of the operation, the surgeon then makes the final determination of the best type of urethral reconstruction. The variety of urethral repairs should have been discussed with the patient and parents in advance of surgery. Frequently the surgeon is able to share recommendations for his or her preferred procedure at the office visit; however, final determination is made at the time of surgery when the quantity and quality of tissue is definitively assessed.

I like to think of urethral reconstructions as coming in four different varieties. There are dozens of names for the different operations but the four underlying principles of repair of the urethra remain the same. Here is a description of these four general approaches to urethral reconstruction:

### 1. Advancing the existing urethral tube to the true apex of the glans.

This technique is often employed in cases of mild hypospadias when the meatus is located at the coronal sulcus or within the glans. The urethral tissue must be very robust and elastic for this to work well. If chosen appropriately, this type of repair has the least risk of complications. A popular operation in this category is the MAGPI Procedure.

Fig. 12

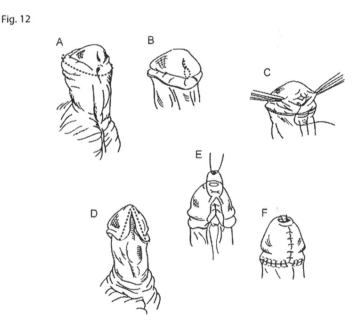

*Figure 12: MAGPI Procedure, which is a common urethral advancement repair. (Source: Kelly Carter)*

## 2. Tubularizing the existing urethral plate

This technique requires a healthy urethral plate. The urethral plate is the strip of soft pinkish tissue on the underside of the penis that is located in the space between the hypospadiac meatus and the apex of the glans where the urethral opening would ordinarily be positioned. If this tissue is wide enough it can be turned into a tube with little difficulty. This is often called a Duplay Tube. I often help parents visualize this procedure by asking them if they have ever used one of the combination straw/spoons provided by 7-11 for drinking a Slurpee (see figure 13). If you bend the edges of the spoon portion together, you create a natural extension of the straw. This is exactly how the urethra is reconstructed in this technique.

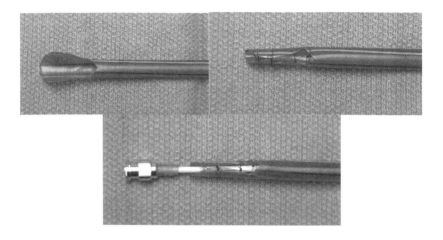

*Figure 13: 7-11 Straw Demo. A) The Slurpee Straw/Spoon. B) The "tubularized" spoon to created the urethral extension. C) The "neourethra" with a small white tube inserted to simulate the post-op catheter. (Source: Dr Bill Kennedy)*

If the urethral plate is not wide enough to make a tube in this fashion, a variation of the procedure can be performed in which the urethral plate has a deep vertical incision made in the mid-portion. This allows for greater width of the plate at the time of reconstruction. This modification in the tubularization procedure is commonly referred to as the Snodgrass Procedure after the surgeon who popularized its use (see figure 14).

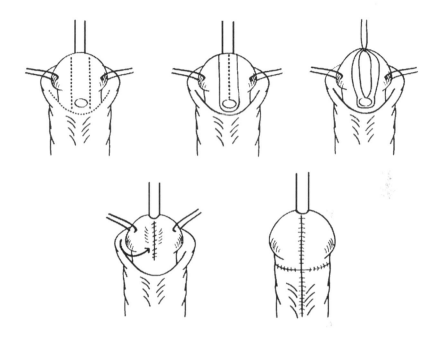

*Figure 14: Diagram of the Snodgrass modification in which a vertical incision is made in the middle of the urethral plate to allow for greater width of the tissue in making the tubularized urethra. (Source: Kelly Carter)*

Duplay Tubes and Snodgrass Procedures are commonly used to repair hypospadias at the mid and upper portion of the penile shaft. Occasionally it is also utilized in penoscrotal hypospadias if the tissues of the urethral plate are very healthy (see figure 15).

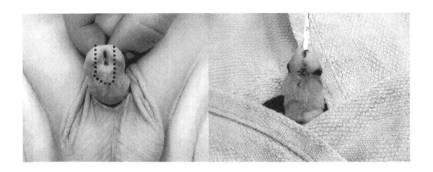

*Figure 15: A) Example of a Duplay Tube repair where the blue dots represent the urethral plate tissue that will be tubularized. B) Completed surgery with catheter in place for healing. (Source: Dr Bill Kennedy)*

### 3. Incorporating vascularized skin onto the urethral plate

This technique is often utilized in the more moderate and severe forms of hypospadias. The skin that is "patched" on to the urethral plate maintains its original blood supply. Rotational and Island Pedicle Flaps are the two most popular ways of performing this technique. The rotational flap is often called a Flip Flap procedure and skin from the lower portion of the penile shaft is rotated in much like a trap door over the urethral plate to create the tube. In an Island Pedicle Flap, the inner tissue of the foreskin is left attached to its original blood supply and then completely mobilized to patch onto the urethral plate (see figure 16). These procedures are intricate and require delicate handling of the tissue by an experienced surgeon. When performed properly they yield very good results, but do have a higher incidence of complication given the complexity.

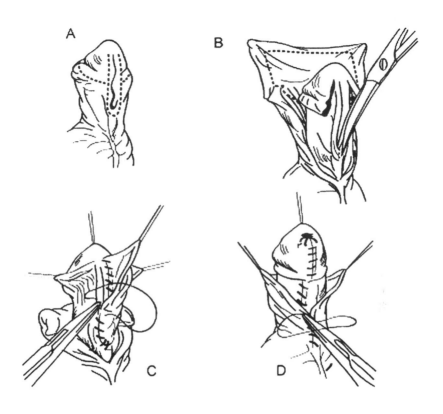

*Figure 16: Island Pedicle Procedure, which is a commonly used in more severe cases of hypospadias. (Source: Kelly Carter)*

## 4. Free grafting of tissue to create the urethra

When there is a shortage of appropriate tissue on the penis to use for urethral reconstruction, occasionally additional sources of tissue may be obtained from distant sites and used to reconstruct the urethra. This technique is most frequently used when prior surgeries have failed and no local tissue is adequate for reconstruction. Free skin grafts from other hairless portions of the body (often the forearm) or buccal mucosa (inside lining of the mouth) are utilized. These techniques are the riskiest of the urethral repairs as they rely on the ingrowth of adequate blood supply for long-term success.

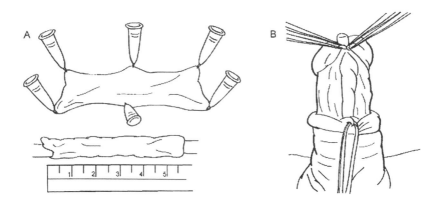

*Figure 17: A) Free Graft of Buccal Mucosa used to fashion a urethral tube. B) The buccal mucosal tube attached to native urethra and brought to top of penis. (Source: Kelly Carter)*

## Strategy for Complex Cases

Occasionally both the hypospadias and the chordee are so severe that a one-stage procedure to repair is not possible or advisable. Frequently there is an element of penoscrotal transposition in which the scrotal tissue is not entirely below the penile shaft. In the case of transposition, the scrotal tissue flanks the penile shaft and often extends superior to the shaft. These are the most complex cases of hypospadias and are often of the scrotal and perineal variety (see Figure 3). Boys that have this category of hypospadias are often referred to as having ambiguous genitalia at birth. Chromosomal analysis is often required to confirm the male sex before any discussion of surgery is appropriate (see figure 18).

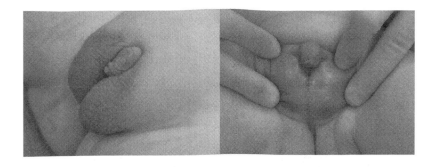

*Figure 18: A) Side view of boy with scrotal hypospadias, severe chordee, and slight penoscrotal transposition. B) View of same child demonstrating scrotal location of the urethral meatus . (Source: Dr Bill Kennedy)*

In these complex cases, the surgery is often staged so that the severe chordee and penoscrotal transposition are corrected in the first surgery. The correction of the penoscrotal transposition is referred to as a scrotoplasty. The urethral meatus is often brought to the penoscrotal junction at this first surgery as well. The tissues are left to heal (6 months) and develop a robust blood supply after this extensive mobilization (see figure 19).

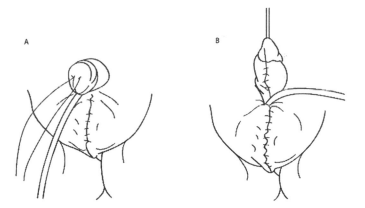

*Figure 19: Two views of patient after the first stage of a planned two stage procedure. The chordee has been corrected and scrotoplasty performed to correct the transposition. (Source: Kelly Carter)*

In the planned second stage of the reconstruction, the creation of the urethral tube from the penoscrotal junction to the tip of the penis is completed. This is performed in the same way as the tubularization technique described earlier. The tissue used to create the urethra is the foreskin that was rotated to the underside of the penis in stage one to correct the severe chordee. Now that it has had the chance to heal and develop good blood flow, it can be mobilized again to make the urethral tube (see figure 20).

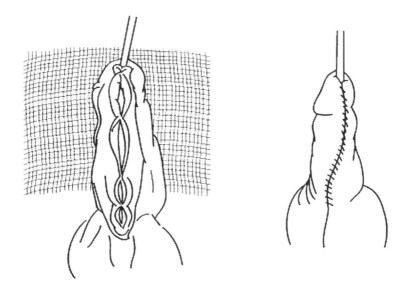

*Figure 20: A) Tubularization of the new urethra from transferred skin at the time of the first surgery. B) Tubularization complete and external skin closed on top to recess the urethra in the shaft of the penis. (Source: Kelly Carter)*

## Foreskin Preservation

In cultures where circumcision is common, very often little attempt is made to preserve or reconstruct the foreskin. Patients and parents should be aware that techniques do exist to successfully reconstruct the foreskin at the time of hypospadias surgery. It is often not advised as the foreskin may be needed for correction of moderate and severe chordee or may be required for a flap to reconstruct the urethra. Foreskin preservation is most successfully performed in cases of mild or moderate hypospadias with mild chordee (see figure 21). If foreskin preservation is culturally important to the patient and parents, it is appropriate to discuss this at the time of surgical planning. When this is not advised by the surgeon, the patient or parent should have a valid reason for this request.

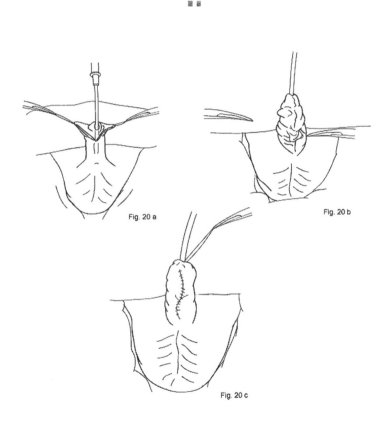

Fig. 20 a

Fig. 20 b

Fig. 20 c

*Figure 21: A) Mild hypospadias for consideration of foreskin reconstruction. B) Tubularization complete of the urethral reconstruction. C) Foreskin reconstruction complete. (Source: Kelly Carter)*

## Post Operative Care

*Please see the example of post-operative instruction that has been included at the end of the book.*

Perhaps just as important as the surgery itself is the post-operative care the patient receives during the healing phase. All surgeons have individualized protocols for the care of their patients. They usually have a rationale for the recommendations that they make. This includes bandages, need for catheter, use of antibiotics, use of bladder spasm medications, and length of time with catheter. It is never too early to ask about the post-operative care plan. Depending on the severity of the hypospadias and the type of surgery performed, the post-op protocols may even change for the same surgeon. The anticipated post-operative plan may impact which date the patient and parents choose to have the surgery performed. Parents may need to plan time off from work to care for the child with a catheter. Often grandparents may help supplement the care of parents. Always ask the surgeon for a printed copy of their post-op instructions so that you may read them and become familiar with them before the surgery. It is very difficult to hear these complex plans for the first time immediately after surgery.

## Bandages

There is no right or wrong bandage to be used in hypospadias surgery. Each surgeon chooses a bandage based on their successful experiences in certain situations. Bandages may vary from surgical skin glues (i.e., Dermabond) to compressive bandages of various types. All surgeons will explain to you the care of the bandage and timing of removal or replacement. The purpose of most bandages is to protect the fresh incisions from contamination and possibly provide pressure to minimize bleeding and swelling.

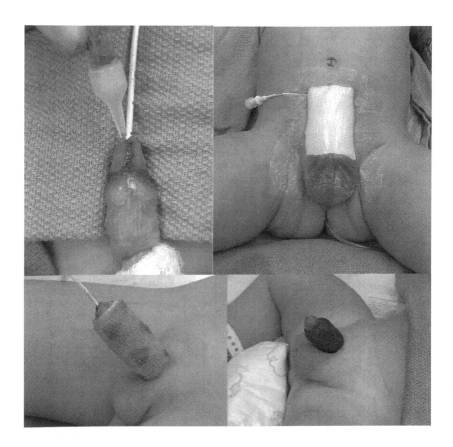

*Figure 22 A) Skin glue applied to surgical wound as a bandage. B) Compression dressing using tegaderm and gauze to fix penis firmly against the abdominal wall. C) Circumferential pressure bandage with coban on patient with catheter reinforcing original bandage. D) Compression bandage with coban with no catheter. (Source: Dr Bill Kennedy)*

## Role of Post Operative Catheters

Most surgeons use a catheter as part of their post operative care plan. The catheters may be held in place by either a stitch or an inflatable balloon within the catheter (Foley Catheter). The reason for the catheter is to divert the urinary stream through the tube so it does not immediately flow through the urethra.

The newly reconstructed urethra would be at considerable risk to develop leaks if a forceful stream of urine were to flow through it immediately after surgery.

Occasionally no catheter is left after surgery. This is usually the case in which the urethral reconstruction is short and a multiple layer closure of the urethral tube with very healthy tissue is achieved. Even in cases such as this, some surgeons always opt to leave a catheter as post-operative swelling of tissue may prevent the patient from urinating.

How long the catheter is to remain in place may vary dramatically from patient to patient and surgeon to surgeon. The shortest duration of a catheter is usually 2-3 days when they are left only as a precaution for urinary retention after surgery due to tissue edema (swelling). When catheters are left to allow the urethral reconstruction to heal, these may stay in place anywhere from 7 to 21 days. The complexity of the repair and the health of the tissues are usually the two most important factors in this determination.

The catheter in younger boys is allowed to drain directly into their diaper. Depending on the style of catheter used, some surgeons advise parents to use a double diapering technique. If this is to be done in the case of your son, be certain that the recovery room staff instruct you on the technique before going home. Older potty trained boys undergoing repairs requiring catheters may also use pull-ups for convenience. In other cases, the catheter may be allowed to drain to a urinary drainage bag that is fastened to the patient's leg. This is usually the case only in boys cooperative and mature enough to manage the drainage bag. The safest and most common drainage method in youngest boys is directly into the diaper as no portion of the catheter is visible or able to be accidentally pulled on. <u>The only activities universally not permitted when a catheter is in place are baths and swimming</u>.

On occasion, especially in older patients undergoing revision surgery, a supra-pubic tube may also be left. This is a tube that directly enters the bladder through the abdominal wall and drains the urine. When urinary diversion (no urine flowing through the penis) is needed for lengthy periods of time, this is a preferred method of drainage. The supra-pubic tube may also attach to a drainage bag fastened to the patient's leg. The benefit of the supra-pubic tube in very complex surgeries is that it may easily be capped to allow for a trial at urinating. If the child is not able to urinate, then it may be easily opened and bag drainage resumed.

## Medications

There are three classes of medications that may be used in the postoperative period.

### Pain Medications

Every patient should be sent home from the hospital with a plan for post-operative pain management. This may include a combination of prescription medications (such as acetominophen with codeine or hydrocodone) and over the counter medications (such as ibuprofen). Depending on the use of regional anesthesia (nerve blocks) during surgery, the immediate need for these medications may vary in patients. Be sure that the surgeon and staff explain the appropriate dosing and timing of all medications to be used.

### Antibiotics

Some surgeons elect to use prophylactic or preventative dosing of antibiotics to avoid urinary tract infections while the catheter is in place. This is generally a once a day dosing regimen. Be certain of the plans at the time of discharge.

### Bladder Antispasm Medications

Some children have sensitive bladders and the urinary catheter may provoke spasm in the recovery phase. A good indicator of whether your child is having spasms is the onset of sharp and sudden pain which resolves rather quickly. Sometimes there may even be urine flowing around the outside of the catheter in addition to through it when a forceful spasm occurs. Once again, surgeons have different protocols for how they use these medications in the recovery phase. Be sure you understand the indications for these medications before leaving the hospital and the dosing schedule if prescribed.

## Post-Operative Complications

Hypospadias surgery is difficult to perform successfully. The surgical principles of repair are all very intuitive and make it appear, on first glance, to be an easy operation. It is not a life-threatening surgery. In the majority of cases, a healthy boy is able to have surgery performed as an outpatient procedure. This, however, is where the simplicity ends. The tissues are delicate, the operative field is quite small and the post-operative care is challenging given the healing environment is often the inside of a young boy's diaper. Successful surgery requires a skilled surgeon, an experienced surgical team, and meticulous follow-up with the patient and family. Even with the best of care, complications can still occur. Let's explore these complications by breaking them up into those that occur early on in the recovery and those that occur after several months.

## Short-Term Complications

**Bleeding**. This is the most common problem after hypospadias surgery. Although common it rarely is to the degree that would require blood transfusion. Most post-operative bleeding is detected in the recovery room and is corrected before the patient leaves the hospital. The standard treatment strategy for early post-operative bleeding is to place a pressure dressing (if one had not been previously employed) or to reinforce the current pressure dressing if it had come loose. Examples of pressure dressings appear in figure 22. In rare situations the patient may need to return to the operating room to have the bleeding controlled by either placement of a stitch or to evacuate a hematoma (blood clot) that may have formed under the skin. Large hematomas may cause wound breakdown or tissue asymmetry (unevenness).

If new bleeding occurs once the patient is at home, the parents should contact the surgeon immediately. Instructions should have been provided with the post-operative instructions. Often parents may be asked to apply some pressure at home to see if the bleeding will stop. If the bleeding cannot be effectively controlled through simple maneuvers described by the surgeon, then a return to the hospital or clinic for a complete assessment may be required. If your child is wearing diapers, always keep the bloody diapers that you have changed and bring them back with you. This will enable the surgeon to better assess the degree of bleeding.

**Infection**. This is a less common complication but often occurs in the early postoperative period (2-5 days after surgery). Some signs of infection may be persistently high fever, increasing redness of the tissues, worsening tenderness to gentle touch, or foul smelling, cloudy urine. If infection is suspected, the surgeon needs to be contacted and the patient must come in for evaluation. Urine and wound cultures may be necessary. The patient will often have treatment strength antibiotics started while results of the culture are pending. Untreated infections can lead to rapid breakdown of the healing tissues.

**Meatal Stenosis**. This is a narrowing of the new urinary opening at the tip of the penis. It can occur for several reasons among which are a tight glans reconstruction or irritation or infection at the tip of the penis. Treatment of meatal stenosis may include in-office dilation of the urethra and application of topical corticosteroid ointment. If meatal stenosis is severe, it may require surgical revision of the opening at a future time when the tissues are more stable. Typically it will be performed not earlier than 6 months after the initial operation. Meatal stenosis is often determined by a significantly narrowed urinary stream and straining of the young child to urinate.

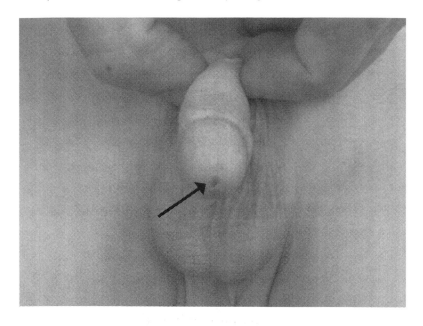

*Figure 23. Meatal stenosis at 6 months after initial hypospadias repair. The arrow indicates the narrowed opening at the tip of the glans penis. (Source: Dr Bill Kennedy)*

**Ischemic Skin Flaps.** This is a rare immediate complication in cases of moderate and severe hypospadias repair in which large amounts of skin mobilization have occurred. Occasionally the blood supply to the skin is compromised and the skin does not survive. Treatment of this complication may require removal of the non-viable or infected skin. Frequently conservative care with protective dressings or antibiotic ointment is performed. Often skin from the surrounding areas slowly grows in to cover the affected region. If any surgical revision is needed, it is best to wait a minimum of 6 months for the tissues to adequately heal before performing the surgery.

## Long Term Complications

### Urethral Fistula

This is the most common long-term post-operative complication of hypospadias surgery. The problem is detected by the patient or parent observing the boy urinate. At the time of urination, a drip of urine from the undersurface of the penile shaft or a second urinary stream may be seen. If a second stream is observed, it can be directed in an entirely different direction than the dominant urinary stream. Frequently young boys will complain of urinating outside the toilet or even on their pants when a fistula is present. Figure 24 shows two young boys with single fistulas detected at the time of potty training.

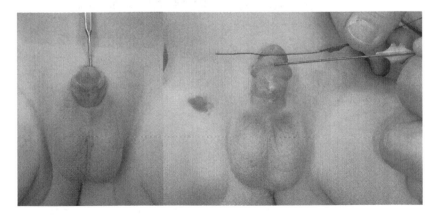

*Figure 24: A) Urethrocutaneous fistula on the undersurface of the penile shaft after initial hypospadias repair. B) The probe indicates small red opening through which urine leaks. (Source: Dr Bill Kennedy)*

The incidence of post-operative fistulas is directly proportional to the length of the reconstructed portion of the urethra. The longer the surgically created tube, the higher risk of fistula formation. Rates of fistula formation in the post-op period range from 2% in cases of mild glandular hypospadias to 20% in the severe cases with an initial urethral opening below the scrotum (perineal). (See Figure 25).

If a urethro-cutaneous fistula is seen in the early post-op period, patient and parents are advised to wait 6 months before making a decision to repair. This recommendation is made as approximately 50% of early fistulas spontaneously close within 6 months after the surgery. Operative repair for fistulas can range from fairly simple surgeries that require no catheter when the fistula is small and the tissues are healthy (see figure 24) to major revision of the hypospadias repair if the fistula is large, tissues are scarred or the location is problematic (see figure 26).

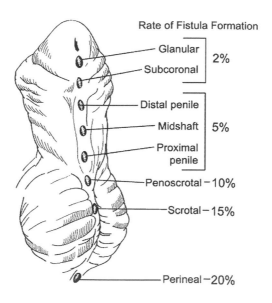

*Figure 25: Rate of fistula formation shown in relation to the initial degree of hypospadias. (Source: Kelly Carter)*

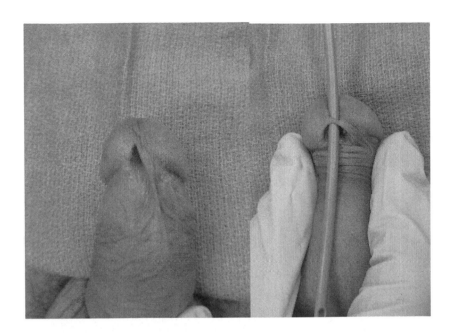

*Figure 26: A) Large fistula located at the subcoronal sulcus. B) Catheter demonstrating fistula and the need to redo the entire glans repair. (Source: Dr Bill Kennedy)*

**Scar Tissue Formation.** Scar tissue can occur at two distinct portions of the repair. The long vertical (length of penis) stitch lines can form scar tissue and result in keloid formation (a specific type of scar tissue). If there is a family history of keloid, then this should be watched for in the early post-operative period. Frequently the early signs of keloid will appear in the first 3 months. If caught early, keloid will often regress with the topical application of a corticosteroid cream such as hydrocortisone. This should be done under the supervision of the surgeon. If you see signs of keloid formation in between scheduled visits, contact your surgeon to address the issue sooner. If keloid is left to mature, it may no longer respond to simple topical treatment and may require revision surgery.

Scar tissue that forms within the newly reconstructed urethra is referred to as a urethral stricture. If a stricture is found in the early post-op period it may respond to dilation therapy. As time progresses, scar tissue becomes more permanent and may require a telescopic (cystoscopy) procedure in which the scar tissue is obliterated or incised. This is often done with a laser. If the scar tissue is very rigid, it may ultimately require open surgical excision and patching with a skin graft. Urethral strictures are usually discovered more than a year after the initial surgery. Young boys who have strictures often report straining to urinate, fine caliber (thin) urinary stream and longer than normal time to finish urinating. All boys with hypospadias repairs should be seen after they are potty trained to assess the caliber of their urinary stream. This may be done by watching them urinate or having them perform a noninvasive test called a uroflow. Cystoscopy or an x-ray test of the urethra may be needed to confirm the diagnosis of a suspected urethral stricture.

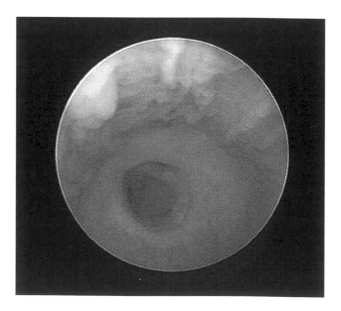

*Figure 27: Urethral stricture confirmed by cystoscopy. Note the concentric narrowing and blanched tissue of the stricture. (Source: Dr Bill Kennedy)*

**Late or Recurrent Curvature.**

Recurrent curvature is a rare long-term complication that may require additional surgery when the child is older. Sometimes the artificial erection during the initial surgery at a young age does not fully uncover the presence of penile curvature. It is only later when the child grows and his erections become more robust and sustained, that this curvature is observed. (see figure 28) Late curvature may occur for two reasons: A) scar tissue formed on the long vertical suture line of the penile shaft, or B) disproportion of the corporal body length only noticed with penile growth. Scar tissue at the skin level can simply be excised. Corporal disproportion needs to be addressed by shortening the longer side of the corpora with a surgery as previously described in figure 10. If the curvature is only very mild, some patients and parents may elect to wait until puberty and let the patient himself make the decision as to whether the curvature is painful or affects sexual function.

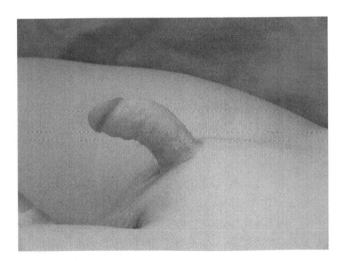

*Figure 28: Reccurrent curvature after initial hypospadias repair.*
*(Source: Dr Bill Kennedy)*

## Urethral Diverticulum

Fortunately, urethal diverticulum is a very rare complication of hypospadias repair. It occurs most commonly in the moderate and severe forms of hypospadias where an extensive neo-urethra has been created from pedicle grafts or free grafts. Since the reconstructive urethral tube lacks the muscular support (bulbospongiosal muscle) of the native urethra it is more prone to dilation over time, especially in an area just before a stricture. Signs of a urethral diverticulum in a potty-trained patient may be swelling of the shaft of the penis with voiding, continued drainage of urine from the urethra post void, and recurrent urinary infections from stasis of urine in the diverticulum. Diverticulum can be confirmed by either x-ray imaging tests or direct visualization with cystoscopy. Uretrhal diverticuli are repaired quite successfully with surgery to remove the excess urethral tissue. Catheters are always required with these surgeries.

## Cosmetic Issues.

Perhaps the most difficult post-operative issues to address after hypospadias repair are those of a cosmetic nature. We all hope for superior outcomes after surgery; however, this can never be 100% guaranteed. All tissues heal in different ways. The skin may react to suture material used by forming skin bridges or suture sinuses. The skin may become asymmetric due to the effects of early infections, scar tissue or large bruise. Frequently what appears to be a major cosmetic issue in the relatively early post op phase improves greatly with growth. Therefore it may be recommended that surgical revision is not immediately needed. If, however, the cosmetic defect gives rise to recurrent skin infections, then earlier repair may be appropriate. Below are some examples of post-operative issues of a more cosmetic nature.

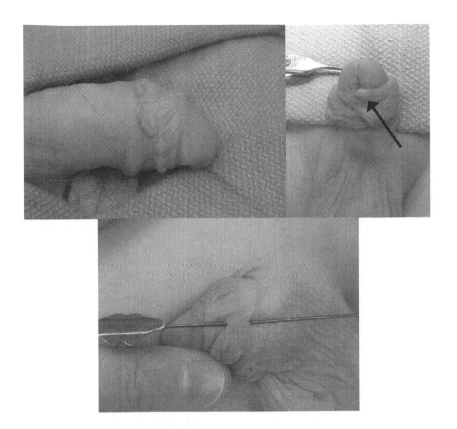

*Figure 29: A) Multiple skin tags around the suture line.. B) Epithelial Inclusion cyst at the site of the subcoronal sulcus C) Suture sinus visible at the suture line. A small probe demonstrates the tunnel of skin that formed around a suture before the suture dissolved. (Source: Dr Bill Kennedy)*

# Chapter 4. Caring for Your Child

*By Genevieve Kilman*

**Summary**

This chapter is about caring for your child and yourself emotionally and physically as you cope with his diagnosis and go through medical appointments and possibly surgery. You will notice that several times I write about the importance of taking care of yourself and your own coping process. Be patient with yourself as you take time to accept the diagnosis, learn how and what you want to share with others, and make medical decisions. Your child will look to you to learn coping and self-acceptance. Children are not easily fooled by your words, but instead pick up on your body language and the emotions behind your words. So please, take the time to take care of yourself and get yourself to a place where you are able to help your child.

**Accepting the Diagnosis**

Every new and expectant parent hopes for a healthy child. Many people when asked, "Are you hoping for a boy or girl?" will answer, "We don't care as long as the baby is healthy." When a child is born with hypospadias, many conflicting emotions can affect how the parents cope with and eventually accept the diagnosis. It is extremely important that as a parent you come to accept your child for who he is and see what a wonderful and beautiful person he is. It is important to do this so you can then help your child cope with his diagnosis. Think of it as the advice you get when riding in an airplane, before securing the oxygen mask on your child, you must secure your own first.

## Grieving

You will go through a process of grief. You will grieve the loss of the child that was to be, the loss of "easy" parenting, the loss of what you had hoped for. If there is more going on with your child than hypospadias, it could mean you may lose the dream of having biological grandchildren. Sometimes, depending on the severity of the hypospadias, you may lose income due to necessary time away from work to take care of your child. Some friends or family may not be as supportive as you would like them to be and so you may have that loss to grieve as well.

Elisabeth Kubler-Ross described five stages that people go through when dealing with death and dying. Her model outlines the five stages of grief that can also be clearly observed in people who are going through any type of loss. Here are the five stages: 1. Denial, 2. Anger, 3. Bargaining, 4. Depression, 5. Acceptance.

You can be in more than one stage at once. Just because you feel like you have dealt with the one stage doesn't mean you are done with it forever. As your child grows and changes, you may grieve again over the loss of what your child is missing out on during that new stage in life. For example, adolescence and coping with your child's physical changes and possible complications from the hypospadias can bring these feelings up again.

Many parents I have worked with reported feeling strong negative emotions when changing their child's diaper or giving him a bath. It was difficult for them to look at their son's penis because it looked so different from what they were used to. This could be especially difficult for parents post-surgery when there is a lot of swelling and most likely a catheter/tube to drain urine from the bladder. Parents often feel sad or guilty for feeling this way. These feelings are all normal and it is important for you to take care of yourself and speak to someone about how you are feeling.

## Sharing the Diagnosis with Family and Friends

### Immediate Family Reaction

The first phase when dealing with a new diagnosis is the crisis phase. Some or all family members suspend normal routine to focus on the crisis. During this time, family is focused on gathering information on hypospadias. Many parents turn to the Internet but it is difficult to find good information. I believe that is why Matt Dorow, as a parent of a child with hypospadias, has been so motivated to publish this book.

New behaviors need to be learned and incorporated into the family routine. Sometimes parents or close family members need to learn how to physically care for the child. Many caregivers will feel the emotional response of guilt, blame, grief, denial, anger, etc. In many ways, the early response sets the stage for how the family will adapt later.

### Reactions outside the Family

Many parents have reported that how the health care professional first told them about their child's hypospadias had a big impact on how they initially felt about it. How much information was given and the words that the health care professional used is important to many parents. What was the nurse or doctor's body language? Did they reassure you? Did they make hypospadias sound more serious or less than it has turned out to be?

Perhaps one of the most painful situations for parents is when they are told that the healthcare professional is unsure if their child is a boy or a girl. Also, if the child is incorrectly identified as a girl and this later is changed, this can be very traumatic for the parents. It is very important that parents in this situation seek out help and talk to someone about their experience. If the parents are able to process what they went through in the early days, they can learn to cope with the diagnosis, accept their child for who he is, and go on to be a wonderful support for their child.

Telling friends, co-workers, neighbors, etc. about your child's hypospadias can be very stressful and scary for some parents. Unfortunately, we live in a culture that does not support people talking about these types of medical issues. Despite the fact that hypospadias is one of the most common birth defects, many people have never heard of it. How much information you want to give people outside of your family is up to you. It will be important for you to identify people you can talk to and rely on. Eventually you will have to teach this same skill to your child so he learns that there are people he can trust to talk to about his concerns. You will quickly learn that some people are more comfortable with and a better support for you than others. Parents I have worked with report that the Hypospadias and Epispadias Association can be a big support. They have information, yearly conferences, online chat rooms, and newsletters that have been very helpful for parents as well as children and men with hypospadias. It will be important for your child to see that it is okay to talk to some people about hypospadias and who the people are that he can trust. This teaches your child that there is nothing wrong with him and talking is not shameful.

**Family Reaction – As Time Goes On**

The second phase of coping with the diagnosis is the chronic phase. During this time, life has to return to your new normal. You learn which friends, co-workers, family, etc. are going to be a support and you cope with the loss of those people who are not able to be as supportive as you need them to be. The ultimate challenge is meeting your child's needs while meeting the needs of all the family members to have a "normal" life. Is the "condition" the centerpiece of your family life or just part of it? A change in your child's function or health may send your family into the crisis phase again. For example, right before or after a surgery may bring up many of the same feelings that you felt right after your child was diagnosed.

## Self Care

There are many books on taking care of yourself. What I have found is that self-care is very personal. For most people, there are general things that will help you cope – getting plenty of rest, exercising, eating well, etc. For others, finding what helps you cope and relax is very personal – it could be a hot bath, a good book, a terrible movie, talking to friends, etc. The important thing is that you take time to take care of yourself. If you do not care for yourself, you will not have the strength to care for your child.

Self-care becomes particularly important when your child is going through surgery. When people offer support, let them help. Many people are not sure what to say or how to help, so give them practical ways they can help you. Some families find it helpful to have friends or family bring them meals at the hospital. If you are going to stay at the hospital for any length of time, you will quickly become tired of hospital food. Other families ask people to help care for their other children, clean their house, throw in a load of laundry, walk their dog, etc. If you are feeling overwhelmed with all that you need to do, make a list and identify which items on the list can be done by other people. Then, when people ask how they can help, hand them the list and tell them to pick an item. Most people feel relieved when given a specific task so they know how to best support you. Your child will need a lot of one-on-one attention and caregiving post-surgery. It is important that you know who you can count on to support you during this time.

On top of the practical support that you will need to take care of yourself, parents often feel they need extra emotional support. It is important that you do not feel guilty for your feelings and instead seek out ways to express those feelings or talk to someone you can trust. Even young children and babies pick up on their parents' emotions. And as your child grows, he will pick up on your feelings and this will affect the way he sees himself. I have worked with parents on rephrasing very negative statements like "When you were a baby, I couldn't stand to look at you" to something more supportive of your child like "I felt very sad when you were a baby because I wanted life to be as easy as possible for you. I loved you and did not want you to have to go through what you have been through. But I know you are beautiful and strong and having hypospadias does not change the person that you are."

Some people may not feel the strong emotions described in the five grief stages. Perhaps for you, you already knew that no one is perfect and having a "perfect" child is not a given. Perhaps you have hypospadias or other medical issues yourself and you are already familiar and comfortable with hospital routines and procedures. Perhaps you do not feel strong emotions when looking at your son's genitals or talking to doctors about surgical options. This does not mean that you do not need to take care of yourself. Even if you have already reached the acceptance stage, there are practical things to consider when your child is having surgery. Do you have someone to help take care of your other children if you have them? Someone to help do laundry, cook a meal, or help around the house? If not, can you hire someone to help you? Would it be helpful to speak with the hospital Social Worker about setting up supports for yourself?

## Overall Strategies for Helping Your Child Cope

- Here are some tips for overall coping. Healthy self-esteem is a child's armor against the challenges of the world. These tips help build your child's self-esteem and self-acceptance.

- PLAY with your child!
- Your child will pick up on your body language, tone, facial expression, etc. What are you "saying" to your child without saying anything?
- Put on your own oxygen mask before putting on your child's – get the help you need.
- ❋ Have an open and honest relationship with your child.
- Include your child in healthcare discussions when he is old enough.
- ❋ When you feel good about your child, tell him.
- ❋ Praise your child often – be specific in your praise.
- ❋ When giving your child feedback, do not criticize him as a person. Focus on behavior needing improvement.
- Teach your child how to make good decisions.
- ❋ Rehearse with your child how they will respond to others teasing him.
- Encourage your child to treat others as he wants to be treated.
- Laugh with your child and teach him to laugh at himself.
- Encourage your child to develop hobbies and interests.
- Encourage your child to form relationships with all types of other children.
- Teach your child to assert his needs.
- Remember – your child is always listening to what you say, how you say it, and what you do!
- Teach your child to be responsible for his actions by being responsible for yours.
- Listen, listen, and listen some more!

**Navigating the Medical System**

While neither the condition nor the complications are life-threatening, no one wants to subject their child to multiple surgeries. Therefore, to reduce the likelihood of complications requiring further surgery, take great care when selecting the surgeon and the surgical team. Remember that the team is just as important as the surgeon. It is the team members who handle and clamp the sensitive tissue; and the team members who educate you, the parent, on how to perform post-operative care. Thus, the quality of the team has a direct impact on the success of the surgery itself.

The one tip I hear most from parents about navigating the medical system is to make sure that you are comfortable with the person or people who are caring for your child. The thought of your child going through surgery will be very scary and anxiety-provoking for most people. It is important that you trust the surgeon and the staff s/he works with. It is also important that you understand what your options are and what the medical plan is. You will want to be sure of your choices as your child grows. Some parents will chose surgery and some will not. Dr. Kennedy's chapter talks more about this.

Here are some tips for gathering information and keeping it together:

- I have noticed that the urologists I work with usually draw pictures to explain surgery to families. Bring blank sheets of paper with you to the appointment and ask the doctor to draw a picture for you as he or she explains what he or she plans to do.
- Gather as much information as you can from the staff – what to expect before, during, and after surgery.
- Now is the time to ask the surgeon any questions you have – remember there is no such thing as a silly question!

- Try to write down your questions before the appointment. When the doctor answers your questions, jot down notes so you remember what he or she said.
- Remember to ask about post-surgery care. Will your child have a catheter (tube to drain his pee)? Will your child have a bandage on his penis? If yes, when does that need to be removed? Will he be in pain? What pain medications will he be given in hospital and what should you give him at home?
- Ideally, both parents should be at the appointment, but if this is not possible, bring a second person with you to the appointment. It is helpful to have someone there to double check information with later.
- Most hospitals have websites that provide helpful information on parking, visitors, what to expect the day of surgery, what to bring to the hospital, etc. Some even have operating room online tours or provide information about getting a tour in person.
- Some parents want to have all of their child's medical information on file at home. You have a right to request any clinic notes, test results, surgery reports, etc. Some hospitals charge a fee to make copies of reports so it may be best to wait until treatment is finished and request a copy of the chart at that point. Ask the clinic staff how to make this request. Usually you will need to go to patient records, sign a legal form, and pay a fee.
- Keep any pictures, notes, and reports in one place. Some hospitals offer families a book/binder to keep all medical information in one place. You can also buy a folder or binder yourself.

## To Take Pictures or Not?

I have many parents ask me if they should take pictures of their child's genitals before and after surgery. They wonder if some day their child will want to know what they looked like before. I believe you should take pictures. Digital pictures are so easy to take and store in a private way. Your child may or may not want to see these in the future but at least if you take pictures, you are making it his choice later on. Some parents also take pictures to show the healing process post-surgery. This can help you determine if there is more swelling or something to be concerned about. It is also a great visual reminder that your child is healing. Parents are often surprised by how much swelling and bruising there is post-surgery. Remember, your child needs time to heal.

Also be aware that many surgeons will want to take pictures of your child's penis. This allows them to compare pre and post-surgery pictures. It also helps them to document what surgery was done and what it looked like afterwards. The surgeon will not take any pictures with your child's face or use any identifying information if using the pictures for teaching. You have the right to refuse that your child's picture is taken. But remember, they are taking pictures to help your child and other children.

If your child is older, having pictures taken should be his choice. Explain why you or the doctor wants to take the picture and be sure it is ok with your child first.

## Typical Surgical Day

Every hospital has its own specific procedures but most follow this general outline. Your surgeon's clinic should give you information about the hospital's specific schedule, when and where to go, etc. Many hospitals also have helpful information on their websites about what to expect. And many websites have tours that walk you through the day's schedule. The events on the surgery day can be grouped based on what happens pre-op (before surgery), waiting during your child's surgery, and post-op (after surgery.)

## Pre-Op

Check In. You will register your child and let the staff know that you are there by checking in. Some hospitals have you check in at a registration desk and others have you check in where your child will be assessed before surgery.

- Nursing assessment. A nurse will assess your child and make sure he is healthy enough to have surgery. It is important that your child not have a cold, fever, or symptoms of being ill. The nurse will check your child's temperature, blood pressure, weight, height, heart rate, and oxygen level. Your child will also change into hospital pajamas at this time and put on a hospital ID band. Some younger children prefer to have ID bands on their ankles where it will not be in their way while they play. Where this assessment takes place depends on the hospital.

- Waiting, waiting, and waiting some more. Most hospitals will have a waiting room with some toys to help distract your child while he waits for surgery. Many parents are very concerned about this waiting time since their child is likely to be hungry from not being allowed to eat before surgery. Most children cope very well with waiting if they are distracted and allowed to play. Be sure to bring along some favorite toys or books for your child in case the waiting room does not have the type of toys your child likes. Some parents buy something new to help with distraction and this works well for some children.

- Meet the anesthesiologist. This is usually the first time you will meet the anesthesiologist (doctor who is in charge of the sleep medication). He or she will assess your child by asking if they have been ill recently, they will listen to your child's heart and lungs, they will look in your child's mouth, they may ask questions about your child's overall health – Does he snore? Get lots of colds? etc. If your child is anxious about falling asleep, this is the best person you can talk to about how to help ease your child's anxiety. Depending on the hospital, the doctor may offer your child a mild sedative to help him relax or it may be possible for you to go with your child until he falls asleep. Many hospitals offer a flavored mask that will give your child sleeping medicine before they put in the IV. This way, your child does not have to have a needle while awake. If your child is anxious about this part, you can talk to your hospital Child Life Specialist about helping your child cope.

- Last-minute questions for the surgeon. Most surgeons or someone from their team will be sure to check in with you while you are waiting to see if you have any last-minute questions/concerns.

- Operating room nurse. The operating room nurse will introduce him/herself and will most likely be the person to take your child into the operating room when it is ready. The nurse usually asks you the same questions you may have already been asked to double check the information and make sure all of your child's forms are filled out and ready.

- Other staff. Typically there are many people involved in helping care for your child during his surgery. If you are at a teaching hospital, you may meet other staff or you may notice that the doctors have staff with them.

**Family Waiting Area**

While your child is in surgery, you will be instructed to wait in a designated waiting area. Most hospitals allow you to check in to this area and then you are free to leave to make some phone calls or get something to eat. The staff should give you an idea of when to report back to the waiting area. Many waiting areas have space and allow families to eat there. I always encourage families to eat at this time. Chances are, you were so busy with getting your child ready that you may not have eaten anything yet. Some parents choose not to eat before surgery if their child is older and may notice that parents can eat when he can't. You will most likely be feeling anxious during this waiting time but it is important to take care of yourself so when your child is out of surgery you have energy to take care of him. Some children are grumpy after surgery and may need a lot of attention.

**Post-Op Recovery Room**

The doctor or someone from his/her team will usually see you in the waiting room to discuss how the surgery went before you go to see your child. When your child's surgery is done and he is settled in the recovery room, staff will allow you to see him. This can sometimes take a while and can be very difficult for parents as they anxiously wait to see their child. Some children take a long time to wake up from the anesthesia and might just be taking a long nap. It does not mean anything is wrong if staff take a while to call you to the recovery room. Some hospitals have a policy that only one parent is allowed into the recovery area due to the small space. If possible, I think it is best that both parents are in the recovery area so they can get the post-surgery instructions and ask questions together. The recovery room is usually very busy and noisy. You may hear some children (or parents) crying. Staff try to keep things as quiet as possible for your child but it is a very busy area. Your child will most likely still have monitors that show his heart rate and breathing. He will also have an IV (a very tiny tube in his hand, arm, or foot that staff can use to give him medication or fluids. An IV is not a needle – the needle is used to insert the IV and then taken out and the tube remains in place). Your child will stay in the recovery area until he is more alert and able to drink something. Some hospitals also offer popsicles or slushies.

## Outpatient Surgery Discharge

If your child is going home the same day as surgery (most children who undergo hypospadias repairs are able to go home the same day), you will receive discharge instructions while in the recovery room. The nurse will go over the information with you. If your child has a stent or catheter, the nurse will explain how to care for this. If your child has a bandage that needs to be removed in a certain time frame, the nurse should explain this as well. Occasionally the doctor may stop by to see if you have any questions. If you have any major questions/concerns or do not feel comfortable taking your child home yet, you can always ask to speak with a doctor. If your child's doctor is in the operating room and unable to come see you, he will be able to send another doctor from his team to answer your questions. Make sure that you have written instructions on how to care for your child, what pain medications to give, when to take the bandage off, and bathing instructions. Most surgeons recommend that parents give their child 2-3 baths a day in warm water with no soap once the bandage is off to help with the healing process. Many parents I have worked with have been afraid to bath their child and sometimes leave the bandage in place. This can be very harmful for your child since it does not allow his skin to heal. If you are unsure about how best to remove the bandage, ask the nurse or call the clinic for advice.

NOTE: We have included samples of post-surgery care instructions at the end of this book. Make sure that your surgical team provides you with such instructions. Be sure that you know what to do for the most common complications. The three most common that you should know how to react to are bladder spasms, bleeding, and no urine flow.

Bladder spasms are caused by the catheter irritating the bladder itself. A bladder spasm is a sudden and often very painful contraction of the bladder. When it occurs in a young boy, he will often cry out in pain and fear. This will be a scary moment. And then after several minutes the pain will subside. Once a bladder spasm occurs, it will likely occur again at some point during the recovery process. Effective anti-bladder spasm medication does exist (Ditropan, which is Oxybutynin), but your doctor will likely not want to prescribe it until it is necessary. You may, therefore, want to ask for this prescription in advance so that you do not have to return to the hospital or pharmacy should bladder spasms begin.

Bleeding can occur when the cut from the surgery does not close properly. If bleeding continues after you apply pressure to the area for several minutes with a clean washcloth, please contact your medical team.

No urine flow is another common complication. Some clotted blood from the surgery may get lodged in the urethral tube or cather, literally clogging it. This can cause pressure to build in the urethral tube or bladder, or cause urine to "leak" into the abdomen. This must be corrected immediately before the surgical stitches are pulled apart. If your son's diaper remains dry for more than 2 hours, this is an indication that urine is not properly flowing out of the catheter or urethral tube. Please contact your medical team immediately.

Contacting medical staff when such complications actually occur (especially if at night or on the weekends) is much more difficult than getting your questions answered while you are talking to the staff in person at the time of the surgery or during pre-surgery visits.

Be insistent about getting the full post-surgical care instructions in writing before the surgery. It is critical to have these instructions in writing, because if a complication arises later, it is highly unlikely that you will remember everything that you were told verbally. In talking to parents of children where the surgeries did not succeed, several shared with us that the complications were caused by inaction on their part. But the parents had not been fully informed by the medical staff and therefore didn't know what they (the parents) were supposed to do, or that they were supposed to act at all.

As an example, if urine is not flowing from the catheter after several hours, it may indicate a clogged catheter. If treated on the same day, no damage will likely occur. If treated the next day, the surgical stitches may already be irreparably damaged.

We also recommend purchasing the medications that you have been prescribed in the hospital pharmacy. The prices are usually cheaper than commercial pharmacies, you can buy the medications while your child is in surgery so there is no distraction after your child comes out of surgery, and most importantly the hospital pharmacy is more likely to have the infant versions of ibuprofen and acetaminophen (flavored liquid). Also, ask your discharge nurse for several syringe plungers, which will make it easier to administer the medicines orally if you choose not to simply add them to your child's milk or food.

## Staying Overnight

If your child has a more complex surgical repair or is an older child, he may need to stay overnight for monitoring. You will be escorted to the inpatient surgical floor once your child is a little more alert in the recovery room. Most hospitals have a parent sleep bed in the same room as your child so you can stay with him. It is a good idea to pack an overnight bag for yourself with essentials like your toothbrush, soap, toothpaste, etc.

Inpatient Nurse. There will be a nurse who is assigned to looking after your child. He/she or one of the other people involved in your child's care will show you around the unit and answer any questions you may have.

## Inpatient Stay

It will be important that your child gets lots of rest after surgery. The doctor will order pain medication and discuss this with you before your child is on the inpatient floor. For more complex surgeries, your child may have an epidural or a pump that he is able to push a button on to administer medication for pain control. Your doctor will discuss all of this with you before surgery. It is important that your child communicate with you and the staff to say how he is feeling. If he is having a lot of pain, it is important for staff to know this so they can make him more comfortable. Most hospitals have a playroom area where your child can play (if he is able to get out of bed) or you can bring him toys, books, or movies from it. It is also a good idea to bring along your child's favorite things. Children cope better with being in hospital when they are distracted by playing. Some hospitals even have laptops that you can borrow for your child if he is older.

The doctor who comes to see your child during his stay may not be the attending physician. You will meet other doctors from his/her team and they will communicate with the doctor for you. If your child has surgery at a teaching hospital, you will meet several doctors who are all part of the team taking care of your child. These doctors may be at different levels in their training. Your child's care will be overseen by the attending doctor and you can always request to see him/her if you have any concerns. The attending doctor may not always be available to see you right away but will communicate either with the nurse taking care of your child or will send another doctor from the team.

## Discharge

When your child is ready to go home, the doctor and nurse will go over all of the discharge instructions with you. Your child may have his bandages removed before going home but it is likely that he will still have a stent or catheter. The nurse will explain how to take care of this. It is important that you get written instructions on how to care for your child, what pain medications to give, bathing instructions, etc. Review these in detail with the discharge nurse. More than one parent has expressed that a perfectly good surgery was undone because post-care instructions weren't clear, and they (the parents) didn't properly address a complication that appeared post-surgery because they didn't know how.

In fact, it is best to get discharge instructions in writing, and review them with the staff, BEFORE the surgery. That way you can make sure that you get the full information you need, before you even allow the surgery to occur.

A very common complication is a blockage of the catheter. Occasionally, a piece of clotted blood from the surgery will enter and block the catheter. If this occurs, then urine will pass around, not through the catheter, potentially compromising the surgery itself. This is a serious issue which must be dealt with immediately. If at any point during the recovery process while the catheter is still in, your son's diaper remains dry for more than 2-3 hours, contact your medical team immediately. Talk to your surgical team about blockages before the surgery, so that you will you know what to look for and what to do if such a blockage occurs.

Another common complication is bladder spasms. These are caused by the catheter used to maintain the structure of the urethral tube post-surgery. The medication Ditropan can be prescribed to minimize the effect of bladder spasms. When a bladder spasm occurs, the boy will suddenly have a very sharp pain in his midsection and will likely scream out in pain (probably like he has never screamed out before). Until the spasm passes, there is little that can be done to alleviate the pain. It is, therefore, a good idea to discuss bladder spasms with your surgical team before the surgery, so that you can determine whether Ditropan is recommended, and if not, so that you can be aware of the symptoms in case they occur.

## Communicating with Staff

It is important to remember that every person involved in your child's care is trying to help him and your family during this stressful time. Like all jobs, some staff members are better at their jobs and have more interpersonal skills than others. The hospital is a very busy place and staff come into contact with many families throughout the day. Sometimes staff may appear more rushed or less helpful than you would like them to be. It is important that you speak directly to staff and let them know what information you need. Staff are people; like everyone else they will each have their own personality. Some staff you may "like" and others you may not. No matter what, you deserve to be treated with respect and it is your responsibility to also treat staff with respect. If you come across a staff member that you find challenging to work with, try to focus on what your child needs and communicate that to the staff. If you have a concern that staff are not addressing your child's need, be sure to focus on what the issue is, not the staff member. I have heard many families feel upset that they interacted with an unhelpful staff member throughout their child's surgical day. If this is the case, just remember that perhaps that person was having a bad day. Unless you have concerns about your child's care, it is usually best to ignore any staff you may not "like" and focus on helping your child. You can always give feedback to the hospital later about your experience but when your child needs you to be there for him, it is usually best to focus on what your child needs.

## Preparing Your Child for Surgery

This section focuses on talking to your child about surgery if you have chosen that option. As stated earlier, surgery is one option and is not always the choice every parent wants. The most important thing is that you or your child (if he is older) knows what the options are before making that decision.

### Why emotionally prepare your child?

- Research has shown that when a child is given developmentally appropriate information about an upcoming medical procedure, he copes better.
- Surgery without proper emotional preparation can traumatize a child.
- Often times, the child has heard you speaking about the surgery and therefore already has fears and mis-understanding. Talking about it allows you to address his fears.
- Children who are not prepared often regress in the weeks and months following surgery.
- Talking about surgery takes the shame away.
- Talking about surgery lets your child know that it is ok to talk about it.
- Talking about surgery gives your child an opportunity to express his feelings.

### Who can help you prepare your child?

- Child Life Specialists are trained professionals that work in most hospitals. Contact the hospital where the surgery is scheduled and find out if a Child Life Specialist is available to meet with you and your child prior to the day of surgery.
- If you live far away from the hospital or you do not think going to the hospital before the day of surgery works best for your child, the Child Life Specialist

can give you information on how much to tell your child and what to say.

- Many hospitals have websites that have information on different age groups -- what words to use, how much information to give, when to talk to your child, etc. Some websites even have virtual tours you can take with your child.
- Parents and/or people who have had the same surgery may be able to give you tips and pointers. Just be aware that your child may not need to know every detail of that person's experience.

**When should you prepare your child?**

When you talk to your child will depend on several factors:

- Your child's age:
  - Infant/Toddler: Your child is in the here and now, tell him the day before, the morning of, and as things are happening.
  - Preschooler: 3-5 days in advance so your child has time to prepare emotionally and talk to you about surgery.
  - School Aged: At least one or two weeks ahead of time so he has time to prepare.
  - Teenager: Ideally, your teenager should be involved in the decision to have surgery.
- Your child's disposition: does he get anxious when you tell him about appointments ahead of time? Is he the type of child who wants to know every detail or does he prefer not to have much information in advance?
- What has your child heard about surgery? Was he there when you scheduled the surgery? Did your child overhear you talking to friends or family about it?

- Has your child asked you about surgery? This is a big indicator that your child is looking for answers – follow his lead.

Remember…

- Most important thing to remember: Preparation is a process – not a one-time session!
- Be honest! This does not mean that you need to tell your child every detail (or your every fear) about surgery. But you need to give honest answers to the tough questions like, "Will it hurt?" or "Why do I have this?"
- Follow your child's cues: if it looks like your child is overwhelmed with the information, wrap up your conversation and come back to it later.
- You can't fix everything: it is ok for your child to be upset, angry, cry, etc.
- This is your child's body: when possible, include him in the medical decisions.
- Find out as much information as you can so you can answer your child's questions. Try to gather information about what your child will experience with all five of his senses: What will he see, hear, taste, feel, and smell? If you don't know the answer, say "I don't know but I will find out for you."
- It's not just the words you say, it's how you say it. Your child will pick up on your body language cues. Your child will adopt your attitude about surgery. If you are coping well and feel confident, how do you think your child will be?

## How do you prepare your child?

OK, great. I am ready to talk to my child, but now what?

**Ages birth to 2 years**

- Your young child picks up on your emotions. He may not understand all that you are saying, but he can tell when you are upset, angry, frustrated, etc. Talk to your child about your feelings but do not overwhelm him.

- Take care of yourself – how are you feeling about surgery? Surround yourself with friends and family who understand and will listen to you. Ask to speak with a hospital Social Worker for support. (This applies to ALL ages!)

- Use very simple terms when explaining what is happening to your child.

- Even young infants will imitate doctors by putting the stethoscope around their necks- your child picks up more than you think!

- The biggest fear for this age group is separation from parents. Reassure your child that you will be there. If possible, plan to have one parent or close family member stay at the hospital with your child.

- Be calm and patient (it is common for children this age to act out) and maintain the same routine/rules. Children look to rules and consistency to make them feel safe. If you start letting your child get away with everything, he will think, "Something must be really wrong."

- Let your child bring favorite toys, books, blanket, etc. from home. This will give your child a sense of security and control over his surroundings.

**Preschoolers**

- Children this age are magical thinkers: your child may develop misunderstandings about why he needs surgery and what surgery will involve. Encourage your child to tell you what he thinks will happen. Do not laugh at or scold your child for his fears. Instead, tell your child what will happen in simple terms.

- Children have a fear of body mutilation. They often think that the doctor will cut off whatever is not working as it should. Unfortunately, sometimes surgery does involve cutting. Explain in simple terms what the doctor is doing and why. Talk to the medical team about what to expect when your child wakes up – what tubes, drains, bandages, etc. will your child see?

- Your child may assume that he needs surgery because he did something wrong. Reassure your child that it is not his fault and explain why he needs surgery.

- Choose your words carefully. A child this age is typically very literal in thinking. Instead of saying, "They will put you to sleep" (which may remind your child of a favorite pet you put to sleep) say "You will get medicine that will make you take a nap."

- Play with your child. Use a doctor's kit or read books about doctors and hospital visits. Your child will communicate his fears and questions through play.

## School Aged

- A big fear with this age is that he will wake up during surgery. Reassure your child that there is a doctor (anesthesiologist) who is in charge of sleeping medicine and will be in the room the whole time. For a child who likes details, you can talk about all of the monitors that will tell the doctor how much sleep medicine his body needs so they will give him the right amount to make sure he stays asleep and does not feel anything the whole time.

- Another big fear is that his body is not perfect and surgery will cause more scars and damage. Be sure to tell your child why he needs this surgery. Also, remind your child that no one's body is perfect- we all look different. The doctors are trying to help to make sure that his body will work the best that it can.
- Children this age are also afraid of being embarrassed. Tell your child that many children his age have had this surgery and felt the same way. Also, reassure your child that you will advocate for his privacy.
- Your child may become angry or quiet as the surgery time approaches – this is normal. Encourage your child to talk about his feelings
- Get your child to explain back to you what he thinks will happen. This gives you the opportunity to check his understanding and answer questions.
- Friends are important to children this age. Include them (only if this is ok with your child) by talking to them about the surgery (make sure their parents know what is going on). See if your child wants his friends to visit at the hospital, call, or send cards/gifts.

**Teens**

- Most children want to be independent by this age. Surgery can make your child feel dependent on you, staff, other relatives, etc. This can make your child frustrated and angry. Encourage your child to be part of all medical decisions (no matter how small they may seem to you). Give your child control by allowing him to take care of tubes, medications, etc.
- Being away from friends can be very stressful. Talk to your teen about how they want to include (or exclude) their friends. Encourage friends to visit, call, text, skype, etc.

- Be truthful: your child will become angry and not trust you if he feels you are keeping secrets from him.
- Encourage your child to talk about his feelings and his understanding of what is going on. You can also give your child a special book or journal to write or draw his feelings.
- Respect your child's privacy. Reassure your child that it is ok if he wants to talk to the doctor alone. He may have questions that he is too embarrassed to ask in front of you.
- Help your child write down his questions to ask the doctor during appointments.
- Help your child research and connect with other people on the web.
- Your child may have strong feelings about surgery. It is normal for teens to feel very angry one moment and cry about surgery the next.
- Even at this age, familiar objects bring comfort. Encourage your child to bring his favorite book, movie, music, etc.

Your teen may want to be in charge of taking care of his bandages, tubes, etc. after surgery. He may be too embarrassed to have you take care of that part of his body. Make sure he understands how important it is to follow all of the instructions and give him privacy to take care of himself.

Many of the fears – that his body is not perfect, he could wake up during surgery, fear of embarrassment, etc. – are the same as for the fears outlined in the School Aged section above, so please read over those tips too.

A big fear or source of discomfort for this age group is having an erection post-surgically. This is often a physical reaction that your child cannot control. This can be very embarrassing for some teens and equally embarrassing for some parents to talk about. The doctor should be able to tell your child what to expect, what to do to make himself more comfortable, and help him know that this is normal. If your child is sexually active, it is important that he discuss when it is safe to resume sexual activities post-surgery. It is important that your child have someone he can discuss these issues with so that he knows this is normal and he does not end up being uncomfortable (both physically and emotionally) during his recovery.

For teens, it is important to let him know that he can talk openly with the doctor and staff, and what he discusses, if he asks the staff to keep it confidential, will not be told to you, the parents. It is very important that he know that he can discuss personal issues privately with the doctor and staff.

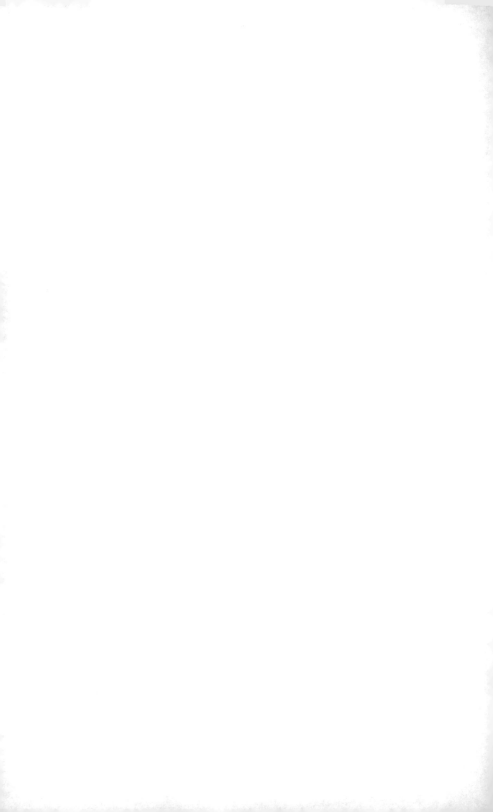

# An Adult's Story

*By Ed Weaver Jr.*

Ed Weaver Jr. is a member of the Hypospadias and Epispadias Association, Inc. (HEA), where he has held the positions of Secretary and President. Born with peno-scrotal hypospadias and chordee, Weaver endured numerous childhood surgeries and repairs, and still faces challenges from hypospadias in his daily life. He strongly advocates for open communication about hypospadias, especially between parents and their sons. Weaver lives in upstate New York.

## Talk to Your Son

On January 14, 1969, I was born into a loving, young, blue-collar family in rural, upstate New York. I have no doubt that my parents were more than just a little shocked, saddened, and anxious to hear that their only son was born with a birth anomaly which they had never heard of before—hypospadias—peno-scrotal hypospadias with severe chordee, to be exact.

I do not recall my parents talking openly with me about my hypospadias. . I believe that they chose this approach because they did not want to draw additional attention to my hypospadias, make me uncomfortable, or risk me developing a negative self-concept. Unfortunately, by not talking to me about my condition, they inadvertently allowed me to develop the negative self-concept that they were likely trying to prevent. I felt alone and scared. I knew that my penis wasn't right, and I thought that

I was the only one in the world like this. I thought there was something wrong with me, not just with my penis.

In hindsight, if my parents had been able to talk to me about it, I would have realized that I was not alone, and there was nothing wrong with me as a person. Unfortunately, that didn't happen. Instead I had to process it all alone, and it has taken me years to do so, and I'm not done yet. It wasn't until I discovered the Hypsospadias and Epispadias Association, Inc. as an adult, that I realized that there were others like me ... and they were good and normal people!

I do not blame my parents or harbor any resentment for my being born with hypospadias; in fact, I feel sorry for any guilt that they have had because I know that this was not their fault. Also, I know that my parents had the best of intentions and supported me to the very best of their ability with something so completely foreign to them.

For me, hypospadias has been much more than just a physical condition—it has had a significant impact on my emotional development and the evolution of my character. I had a series of four surgeries to "fix" my hypospadias within the first five years of my life; unfortunately, my surgical result and the development of unresolved fistulas continue to affect my urinary functioning to this day. Also, I have to sit to pee. As I was growing up, these "differences" made me extremely self-conscious, which in turn developed into an underlying lack of trust of others. On the other hand, I also developed a deep ability to have empathy for others, which is a true gift. As an adult, I've been able to overcome (slowly but surely) the negatives, and embrace the positives.

As parents, you have many factors to consider, and many choices to make, as you determine the best way to respond to this new, unexpected reality. Whether you chose to pursue surgical intervention or not, it is a choice. The best you can do is to:

Educate yourselves about hypospadias, the options available, and your rights.

Openly communicate with your child.

Become a steadfast advocate for your child.

Find support in others who have experienced similar challenges.

All of these are important, but openly communicating with your child is vital!

When you talk to your son about his hypospadias, let him know:

What hypospadias is.

He can approach you if he wants to talk about hypospadias.

That he was born with it, and that he is not alone. Hypospadias is fairly common.

That in addition to talking to you, there are other resources for him to learn about hypospadias and even communicate with others who were born with hypospadias

## Continue to Talk as He Grows Up

Though your son may be very young when he is treated for hypospadias, bear in mind that when he hits puberty, his whole body will grow, including his penis. At this time a fistula or stricture might occur. This is nothing to worry about, as it can be repaired. These repairs are typically performed as outpatient procedures that do not require an overnight stay in the hospital. Remind your son that he should tell you if anything unusual changes in his penis (like the flow of his urine or the point from which it emerges), and then together you can have it assessed and repaired (if that is what he chooses).

Your son will need to be mindful of these possibilities and monitor his health throughout his life. If he does experience a problem and you have not yet told him of his hypospadias, or it has been such a long time since you discussed it that he has forgotten, he will be utterly shocked, scared, and confused. He might be too embarrassed to mention anything to you. That would be a true tragedy, because he would then suffer needlessly and alone.

And in addition to the unnecessary psychological pain, depending upon the complication, a delay in treatment could result in additional medical issues.

I know of a man who went for 30 years without telling anyone that he had a blockage in his penis that made his urine stream veer off to one side, because he was embarrassed about it. When he finally did talk about it (many years later, as an adult), he discovered that the correction for this blockage was simple. He suffered in silence all those years unnecessarily.

## How You Can Help Your Child

From a son's perspective, I believe you as a parent can provide your son with:

Knowledge. Empower your son with age-appropriate information about his hypospadias and make sure he knows that there are others out there like him. As he grows and develops a greater understanding of his hypospadias, he will be better able to advocate for himself and make informed decisions regarding his condition and treatment.

Communication. Talking with your son about his penis, including sex, tends to be an uncomfortable topic for parents, but you can set the stage for open communication at an early age. This will let your child know that this is a safe topic to discuss and he can approach you with any questions that he may have as he develops. Practicing this early in childhood will make conversations much easier as your child enters puberty and transitions to adulthood.

A positive self-image. Your child will look to your lead when establishing his own opinion about his hypospadias. The more you "normalize" his hypospadias, the more you promote a positive sense of self for him.

Support. Connecting your son (and yourselves) with others affected by hypospadias can be truly powerful and reinforce your child's sense of normalcy. This has been one of the most healing things for me – realizing that I am not alone!

# A Parent's Story

*By Matt Dorow*

## Our Son's Story

My wife gave birth to our first son in January of 2009. He was born healthy, happy and with moderate hypospadias. We had no idea what that meant, so we began researching on the internet when we got home. But we could only get very basic information. I am a researcher by nature. And I felt frustrated by the lack of available information.

We were in the San Francisco area at the time, so we scheduled an appointment to see Dr Larry Baskin at UCSF, a highly recommend pediatric urologist in the Bay Area. We were about to move to Brazil for six months (my wife is Brazilian). Dr. Baskin recommended we see Dr. Antonio Macedo, who is based in Sao Paulo, Brazil, and is also a top hypospadias surgeon. We agreed, and Dr. Macedo performed the hypospadias repair surgery when our son was 9 months old. Dr Macedo's team was exceedingly attentive to our son and to us personally, but even so the process was traumatic, watching our infant be subjected to major surgery with general anesthesia. We prayed that our son would only have to experience this once. Unfortunately, those prayers went unanswered. Soon after the surgery, a fistula developed at almost the exact same spot as the urethral opening before surgery.

It was only at that point that my wife and I realized just how difficult this surgery is, and we no longer wanted one of the best surgeons in the world. We would only be satisfied with The Best surgeon (and surgical team) in the world. Our hunt began.

We were far more determined than the first time to find out all that we could. But getting information was no easier. After many months, I stumbled across the Hypospadias and Epispadias Assocation's annual meeting and attended. Suddenly, in a space of 48 hours, I got all the information that I felt I needed. I highly encourage you to attend their conference as well. It will give you far more information than this book ever can.

As for our path, we concluded that Dr. Warren Snodgrass in Dallas was the right surgeon for us. We interviewed him and his team extensively over the phone, as well as other parents that his staff referred us to. We agreed that we would fly to Dallas for a first consult, and then Snodgrass would perform the surgery on the following day if it was warranted.

So, we packed the entire family up and travelled to Dallas for 2 weeks when my son was 19 months old. As planned, we met with Snodgrass and then had the surgery the very next day. The staff was as good in person as they were on the phone. My son had a "complete redo". Snodgrass and his direct team were very attentive to us before, during and after the surgical process. And this time the surgery worked perfectly. We couldn't have been happier.

But even here, there were lessons learned. Snodgrass' team did not give us written post-op instructions. On Day 2 (Saturday), when my son started screaming in pain like we had never heard him scream before, we were scared out of our minds. We frantically called the hospital. 45 minutes later an on-call physician called us back.

She explained that the pain was likely from bladder spasms caused by the catheter. Ditropan could be prescribed. But if we simply waited, there was a good chance that the bladder would adjust to the catheter and the spasms would subside and eventually disappear. Since Ditropan has some side effects, like dryness of the eyes, nose and mouth, she preferred not to prescribe it.

We asked her to prescribe the Ditropan anyway so that if the spasms occurred again, we could begin administering the medicine without delay. She agreed. We picked up the medication and felt much safer. We ended up not needing to administer it.

In hindsight, we would have asked for a full briefing on this and the other common post-operative complications before we left the hospital, so that we would be prepared for them, and know what to do. It seems that most surgical teams, even the best and most experienced, don't focus on this transfer of information to the parents. Therefore, we, as parents, must focus on it. This book, hopefully, will give you enough information to ask good questions.

In the end, the second surgery held. There were no fistulas. The penis was straight and the urethral opening was at the end of the penis. The surgery was a complete success. Our son would be able to pee standing up.

But we knew that our job as parents was not over. The men that I had met at the Hypospadias and Epispadias Association conference made it very clear to me that we needed to tell our son that he was born with hypospadias, so that he would be prepared, and not frightened, if a complication should occur at some point later in life. Just as we wished the surgical team had prepared us for possible complications, so we need to prepare our son.

## My View

Parents have two choices to make:

1. Whether and how to have their son's hypospadias treated surgically.

2. When and how to talk to their son about his condition.

The surgical options today are excellent. While good data have not been systematically collected, the top surgeons claim that they only see complications in about 5% of their first-time surgeries for moderate and severe hypospadias repair, and much less for mild hypospadias repair.

The repair for mild hypospadias is much simpler than that for moderate or severe, and the complication rate for the mild repair is also very low. If a complication does arise from the mild repair, it is usually that the scar tissue at the end of the penis forms a constriction. This is relatively easy to correct.

The visible awkwardness of mild hypospadias is minimal, because the boy will still be able to stand at a urinal. There is a good chance that others might not even notice that there is a difference. So the decision as to whether to repair surgically is not an easy one. As just mentioned, the repair has a very high rate of success, and if a complication does arise it is usually easy to fix. Thus, the benefit of the surgical repair is modest, but the physical cost is low.

The situation for moderate to severe hypospadias is not nearly as benign. The repair is much more invasive. A relatively common complication is a fistula, or hole, appearing along the shaft of the penis where the skin has been closed. A fistula can also be relatively easy to repair. The dead tissue around the fistula is cut out, and a patch of healthy tissue is grafted onto the area. However, if the fistula is near the head of the penis where the new urethral opening is, and cutting out the tissue around the fistula would cause there to be only a thin strip of tissue on the underside of the new urethral opening, then this relatively straightforward method cannot be used because the thin strip of tissue would likely tear. To repair this type of fistula, the penis must be opened and the urethral tube reconstructed from scratch as is done in an initial moderate hypospadias repair ("a complete redo").

The visible awkwardness of moderate to severe hypospadias is very high. The boy will have to sit to pee. The boy will spend his whole life trying to hide this fact from others, affecting his life greatly. The surgical repair, however, is very invasive and the risk of complication is not insignificant. In addition, a quite common complication of a fistula appearing near the head requires a complete redo of the original surgery. Thus the benefit of the surgical repair is high, but the physical cost is also high. Once again, the decision to repair is not an easy one, and the stakes are much higher.

So, what to do? As a parent, do you have the surgery done? And if so, when? And by whom?

In my opinion, the decision of what to do with moderate to severe hypospadias is easier. I recommend the surgery since the benefits are so great. However, great care must be taken in choosing the surgeon.

Mild hypospadias is a closer call. If a boy can stand up to pee at a urinal since his pee shoots forward, others may never notice any difference in his penis, and he may never feel self-conscious about it. Because there is always a false hole at the very tip of the penis anyway, his penis may appear normal to the casual observer. If this is the case, surgical repair may not be worth it.

Chordee, or bending of the penis, often occurs with hypospadias. This bending is often caused by fibrous strands that hold one side of the penis shorter than the other side. Once these strands are cut, which can easily be done during circumcision, the penis usually springs out straight. So, if a boy has mild hypospadias with chordee, I would usually recommend having the circumcision to see if it corrects the chordee. If it does, nothing more need be done. If the circumcision is performed and it is not enough to repair the chordee however, then the more invasive surgery can be initiated, and at the same time the mild hypospadias can be repaired. But in order for this to be possible, the circumcision must be performed by a top pediatric urologist surgeon who has the ability to do the hypospadias surgery on the spot if he/she sees that the circumcision did not resolve the chordee.

As to when to have the surgery, most surgeons seem to prefer to perform the surgery when the baby is between the ages of 6 and 18 months. If the baby is younger than 6 months, the penis is very small and difficult to perform surgery on. Additionally, a baby under 6 months may not tolerate general anesthesia well. After 18 months, babies begin to be more mobile and appear to be more traumatized by the experience of surgery. Before 18 months of age, the baby is relatively immobile, and later in life will not even remember that he had a surgery during this time.

If more than one surgery is required, there is typically at least a 6-month wait between the two surgeries to allow the body to fully heal from the first surgery. For this reason, surgeons often prefer to do the first surgery at or near 6 months of age. This allows them a fairly wide window to perform any additional surgery that might be needed (e.g., to repair a complication that might arise from the first surgery).

## Which Surgeon to Pick?

Mild hypospadias repair is a fairly straightforward surgery. Moderate to severe hypospadias repair is not. The tissue must be very delicately handled. Even if the surgeon does a perfect job, an assistant may incorrectly clamp a piece of tissue damaging the blood vessels. If this occurs, then once that tissue is stitched back it will not form fresh blood vessels and a fistula will appear. So, when you choose a surgeon, you are also choosing his/her surgical team. If any single person on that team makes a mistake, a complication will arise later.

In addition, the nursing staff will be giving information to you as the parent as to how to take care of your child post-operatively, and what complications to look for. If the staff members are not knowledgeable or not communicative, you will miss out on key information that could in the end compromise a perfectly good surgery.

For these reasons, it is vital to seek out a top surgeon and surgical team. Seek out a surgeon who is experienced and located in a facility where hypospadias repair is frequently done. This surgeon will be a pediatric urologist. He or she should be well known for hypospadias surgery. It is important that the surgeon has performed enough surgeries to be comfortable with all the techniques used. The surgeon will not be able to tell exactly how best to repair the hypospadias until s/he begins surgery and sees the condition of the tissue. Since the surgery needs to be done immediately after this assessment, the surgeon needs to be extremely skilled in all of the different surgical procedures so that s/he can use the one that is appropriate for the existing conditions.

Some very experienced surgeons decide to stop operating and move into a teaching role in which they supervise surgery and teach other surgeons. If this is the case for your preferred surgeon, and it makes you uneasy, discuss it with the surgeon. If you are still uncomfortable, ask for a referral to a different surgeon.

There are quite a few top surgeons. Here is just a small sample of pediatric surgeons who are well known for the high quality of their surgeries (as of the writing of this book): Warren Snodgrass in Dallas, Monir Hana in New York, Rafael Gosalbez in Miami, Joao Pippi Salle in Toronto, Larry Baskin in San Francisco, Antonio Macedo in Sao Paolo Brazil, and Bill Kennedy at Stanford. There are many others not on this list. The names above are simply the ones that I know of.

While the surgeons above are all excellent, and their surgical teams all have significant experience and therefore can be expected to follow proper protocol, you must choose the team that you are most comfortable with. Interact with the staff. Which is the most communicative and helpful? Ask for referrals to other parents that you can talk to. Ask the doctor what procedures are used to ensure that the surgical team handles tissue appropriately. Choose the team that you feel gives you the best information in a timely manner.

## Communication

Now that we have discussed surgical repair, let's turn to the even more important topic of communication. It is shocking to me that there isn't more information publicly available about hypospadias. It is, after all, a very common birth defect. And yet, there is almost no information available. Four to six in 1,000 men have it. And yet, do you know anyone who has it? Of course you do, you just don't know exactly who. The fact is that no one talks about it. It occurs in a part of the body that is discussed neither in society nor in family. We don't want to think about it, so we don't talk about it. Unfortunately, this silence has disastrous consequences.

In talking to adult men with hypospadias, their consistent advice to me as a parent was simply that I talk to my son about his hypospadias. Even if his surgical repair proves to be 100% successful, I was advised to explain to my son that he was born with the condition and educate him on the repair, as well as the possible future complications. It's important to do this, because it is very common for a complication to arise later in a boy's life, particularly when he reaches puberty at ages 11-15. It is at this time that the penis (and the body) begins to grow significantly. However, scar tissue does not grow. This can suddenly cause a constriction (and sometimes even a fistula) in the penis.

If a teenager has never been told that he has had hypospadias repair, he may be unaware that this new occurrence (of it taking longer and longer for him to pee, or a hole suddenly appearing in his shaft) is a normal and fixable occurrence. He may be humiliated and not want to talk to you or anyone about it. He may feel that God is punishing him for masturbating (I have heard this quite a few times, because the timing of first masturbations and hypospadias complications occurring can be very close). Whatever it is, he will likely feel very alone and very scared. If you haven't told him about his hypospadias, he may feel like a freak.

If on the other hand, you have told him about his hypospadias, and you have made the penis an open topic, then he will tell you if these complications arise. Then together you can determine how to address them. The repair is often very simple. And the repair is much better than the alternative of suffering in silence.

Another very helpful thing to do is to find other boys with hypospadias that your son can meet. By meeting one or two other boys/men with hypospadias, your son won't feel that he is alone in the world. It may seem silly, but it works. Come to the HEA Conference, or post an ad on Craigslist. A recent such ad in San Antonio, garnered 35 responses. That is 34 more than is needed to let your son know that he's not alone.

# Post-Operative Instructions

**Post-Operative Instructions**

Lucile Packard Children's Hospital
Stanford University School of Medicine

HYPOSPADIAS REPAIR WITH DRAINAGE TUBE

POST OPERATIVE INSTRUCTIONS

Division of Pediatric Urology

(reprinted with permission)

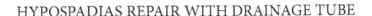

Your son will be discharged home today once he is fully awake and drinking. He has had surgery to repair his hypospadias and he will need some care from you at home to recovery from his surgery. Please see the information and instructions below to help you care for him after you go home.

# PAIN
- **Normal:**
  - o Your child will receive pain medication during and right after the surgery.
  - o He may continue to have some discomfort from the procedure in the first few days after surgery.
- **Things you can do to help with Pain:**
  - o Acetaminophen (*Tylenol*) may be given every 4 hours as needed for pain; check bottle for dosage by your child's weight.
  - o Ibuprofen (*Motrin*) may be given every 6-8 hours as needed for pain instead of Acetaminophen.
  - o *Acetaminophen with Codeine* may be prescribed for the first few days after surgery; afterwards, regular Acetaminophen or Ibuprofen is ok.
  - o *Oxybutynin (Ditropan)* may be prescribed for potential bladder spasms.
  - o **Please call our office (see phone number below) if your child has severe pain even with the pain medications you have been giving.**

# DRESSING AND DRAINAGE TUBE
- **Normal:**
  - o Your son has a clear bandage around or on top of the penis.
  - o He also has a drainage tube placed in the urethra; it is secured by a stitch.
  - o Urine will drain out continuously from this tube into his diaper; the diaper will always be wet.
  - o Your doctor may instruct you to use 2 diapers - with the drainage tube draining between the diapers (double diaper).
  - o **(Check with your nurse)**
  - o Return to clinic in 3-5 days (on ) for dressing removal,

○ **OR**

○ Remove the dressing in 2 days (on ) if it does not fall off on its own.

○ Drainage tube will be in for 10-14 days.

**Things you can do to care for the dressing and drainage tube:**

- If the bandage falls off on its own, it is OK. **No other dressings are necessary**.

- **Please call our office** if the bandage falls off on the same day of surgery.

- After the bandage and drainage tube are removed, you may put some Vaseline around the head of the penis, or directly on the diaper. This can prevent irritation of the penis from the diaper.

- **Please call our office** if you were instructed to remove the dressing at home, but you are having difficulty with the procedure. Sometimes it is easier to remove the dressing if you get the edges wet with a small amount of water.

## APPEARANCE

- **Normal:**

  ○ The penis, head of the penis, and scrotum will appear very bruised, swollen, red, and raw. This will be more noticeable when the dressing has fallen off. This is **Normal and Expected - This will improve in the next few weeks.**

  ○ The stitches will dissolve in a few weeks.

  ○ It is **normal** to have some yellow/green soft material around the stitches.

- **Action: Please call our office if:**

  ○ **There is purulent (pus) drainage from the stitches.**

  ○ **You smell a bad (Foul) odor around the stitches.**

o If the redness near the stitches grows/spreads and extends outward.

o If you see more than one stream of pee when your son pees (urinates) (through fistula opening).

## BLADDER SPASMS
- **Normal:**
  - o Your son may experience bladder spasms with the urinary drainage tube in the bladder.
  - o He may be placed on a bladder relaxant medicine called *Oxybutynin (Ditropan)*.
- **Things to do to help the bladder spasms:**
  - o If *Oxybutynin (Ditropan)* is prescribed, give every 8 hours until the tube is removed.
  - o Possible side effects of *Oxybutynin* include reddening in the face and/or dry mouth while using the medicine.
  - o Constipation may occur with the use of *Oxybutynin*. Give your child plenty of fluids. Our office may also recommend your child start a stool softner, such as Miralax. Give as instructed.
  - o **Please call our office if he does not tolerate *Oxybutynin*.**

## ANTIBIOTICS
- **Normal:**
  - o Your son may be on antibiotics while his urinary drainage tube is in.
- **Your instructions regarding antibiotics:**
  - o If antibiotics are prescribed, give as directed until 3 days after his drainage tube is removed.
  - o **Please call our office if he does not tolerate his antibiotics.**

## BLEEDING
- **Normal:**
  - Dry blood may be seen around stitches.
  - Dried blood and blood-tinged urine may also be seen on diapers.
- **Action to take if there is bleeding:**
  - If there is active bleeding or oozing from the stitches, apply constant gentle pressure with a clean wash cloth for 5 minutes.
  - **Please call our office if active bleeding does not stop after 5 minutes of pressure.**

## URINE OUTPUT
- **Normal:**
  - There may be blood-tinged urine for the first few days.
  - Your son should resume regular urine output; diapers may be changed every 3-4 hours.
  - He may experience slight discomfort with the drainage tube.
- **Action: Please call our office if:**
  - **The drainage tube falls out.**
  - **Diapers are dry for more than 2 hours.**
  - **Abdomen is pushed out (distended) and/or hard.**

## FEVER
- **Normal:**
  - A low grade fever during the first 24 hours after surgery is normal.
  - Encourage fluids and give Acetaminophen for low grade fevers (lower than 101o F).
- **Action:**
  - **Please call our office if there is high fever (higher than 101o F) even after he is given acetaminophen (Tylenol).**

## BOWEL MOVEMENT
- **Normal**:
    - ○ Look for your son to have normal poops (bowel movements); at least one soft stool per day.
    - ○ Acetaminophen with Codeine may cause constipation.
- **Things you can do to help prevent constipation:**
    - ○ Prevent constipation to avoid excessive straining; give plenty of fluids, juices, and vegetables to soften the stool.
    - ○ Regular activities will also help to avoid constipation.
    - ○ If constipated you may start Miralax as directed.
    - ○ Please contact our office or his pediatrician if he has severe constipation

## ACTIVITY
- **Normal**:
    - ○ Normal activity is allowed: quiet play, riding in cars, carseats, strollers.
    - ○ Continue to monitor his activities today due to anesthesia.
- **For the next 2 weeks, avoid activities that may cause oozing from the stitches such as:**
    - ○ Straddling or jumping toys
    - ○ Rough or active playing
    - ○ Sliding down chairs or sofas
    - ○ Wrestling or gymnastics

## BATHING
- **Normal**:
    - ○ Give sponge baths until his dressing and drainage tube are both removed.

- **Things to know about bathing your son:**
  - o Resume regular baths after the dressing and drainage tube are removed.
  - o Avoid long baths for the first 2 weeks to prevent the stitches from dissolving too early.

## DIET
- **Normal:**
  - o Regular diet can be resumed once he tolerates liquids without throwing up (vomiting).
- **Action:**
  - o **Please call our office if your child continues to throw up, and is unable to keep fluids down.**

## CLOTHING
- **Normal:**
  - o It is fine to dress your child in whatever is comfortable for him and for you.
- **Dressing your son:**
  - o May use larger size diapers, and apply tightly to prevent urine leakage from the side of the diaper.
  - o One-piece undershirt is helpful in preventing your son from grabbing the drainage tube under the diaper.

## POST OPERATIVE VISIT:

Your son should return for post-op check in 2-14 days.

Appointment date and time: _____.

Please call _____ the following day to schedule an appointment if you do not have one at the time of discharge from the PACU.

## IMPORTANT PHONE NUMBERS:
- During Regular Business Hours: _____
- During      Evenings,      Weekends      or      Holidays: _____, ask for the Pediatric Urologist on call.

# Contributors

**Matt Dorow** is a father whose son was born with hypospadias. Dorow discovered how difficult it was to find accurate, reliable information about hypospadias. *Hypospadias: A Guide to Treatment* was created as a resource for families in response to his experience. Dorow lives in the San Francisco Bay Area in California.

**Suzan Carmichael**, PhD is an Associate Professor of Pediatrics at the Stanford University School of Medicine. She received her doctorate in epidemiology at the University of California, Berkeley and then served as an Epidemic Intelligence Service Officer in the Division of Reproductive Health at the National Centers for Disease Control and Prevention. She was an epidemiologist with the March of Dimes / California Birth Defects Monitoring Program from 1998-2010. In 2010 she joined the faculty at Stanford. She has published numerous articles related to birth defects risks and maternal and infant health. In particular, she is well-known for advancing current understanding of the etiology of hypospadias, having published some of the largest studies on a variety of risk factors for this outcome.

**Bill Kennedy**, MD is an Associate Professor of Urology at the Stanford University School of Medicine, as well as the Associate Chief of Pediatric Urology at Lucile Packard Children's Hospital at Stanford. He is a practicing pediatric urologist at the Pediatric

Surgical Specialties Clinic at Lucile Packard Children's Hospital. Dr. Kennedy has won many awards in his career, including Compassionate Doctor Recognition from Vitals.com (2010), Best Doctor from Best Doctors in America (2008 - 2011), Patient's Choice Award from MDx Medical in INC. (2009, 2010), Top Urologist from the Guide to America's Top Urologists (2009, 2010), and the Rose Award from Lucile Packard Children's Hospital at Stanford (2009). Dr. Kennedy is board-certified as a pediatric urologist, did his fellowship at Children's Hospital of Philadelphia, his residency at Columbia Presbyterian Medical Center in New York, and received his medical degree from Columbia University.

**Genevieve Kilman** is a Certified Child Life Specialist in the Urology Department at the Hospital for Sick Children in Toronto, Canada. Kilman studied Child Life at Wheelock College in Boston, MA. She completed several internships at Boston's Floating Hospital, The Children's Hospital of Philadelphia, and a trauma treatment and prevention center in Boston, MA. Genevieve has worked as a Certified Child Life Specialist at St. Christopher's Children's Hospital in Philadelphia, The Children's Hospital of Philadelphia, and The Hospital for Sick Children in Toronto, Canada.

**Ed Weaver Jr.** is a member of the Hypospadias and Epispadias Association, Inc. (HEA), where he has held the positions of Secretary and President. Born with peno-scrotal hypospadias and chordee, Weaver endured numerous childhood surgeries and repairs, and still faces challenges from hypospadias in his daily life. He strongly advocates for open communication about hypospadias, especially between parents and their sons. Weaver lives in upstate New York.

Made in the USA
Lexington, KY
29 August 2016